Eating Soulfully
and Healthfully
with Diabetes

Eating Soulfully and Healthfully with Diabetes

Includes Exchange List and Carbohydrate Counts for
Traditional Foods
from the American South and Caribbean

Constance Brown-Riggs,
MSEd, RD, CDE, CDN

iUniverse, Inc.
New York Lincoln Shanghai

Eating Soulfully and Healthfully with Diabetes
Includes Exchange List and Carbohydrate Counts for Traditional Foods
from the American South and Caribbean

iUniverse books may be ordered through booksellers or by contacting:

iUniverse
2021 Pine Lake Road, Suite 100
Lincoln, NE 68512
www.iuniverse.com
1-800-Authors (1-800-288-4677)

This book presents general guidelines for developing a personal meal plan for
people with diabetes. Individuals are advised to consult a physician or other
appropriate health-care professional before undertaking any diet or exercise
program. The advice and strategies contained herein may not be suitable for every
individual. Professionals must use and apply their own judgment, experience, and
training and should not rely solely on the information contained in this publication
when prescribing any diet or exercise regimen.

ISBN-13: 978-0-595-38051-0 (pbk)
ISBN-13: 978-0-595-82421-2 (ebk)
ISBN-10: 0-595-38051-4 (pbk)
ISBN-10: 0-595-82421-8 (ebk)

Printed in the United States of America

We learn to live well
the same way we gain skill
or any art or craft...
by the daily routine of
practice, discipline, and hard work.

Author unknown

This book is dedicated to my family, friends, and patients who struggle daily to manage their diabetes.

Contents

Preface

The intent of this book is to provide a culturally appropriate resource that will facilitate the improvement in outcomes of diabetes in the African American population.

It is well known and supported in scientific literature that much of the morbidity and mortality of diabetes can be eliminated by aggressive treatment with diet, exercise, and new pharmacological approaches to normalizing blood glucose levels. Unfortunately, a wide gap still exists between actual and ideal diabetes care and practice.

African Americans with diabetes are often labeled noncompliant, because they fail to follow nutritional recommendations. A fact that is often overlooked is that these recommendations are unrealistic and culturally insensitive. Furthermore, while there is a plethora of books on diabetes and food counts, there are few, if any, that categorize soul food as a cuisine or include brand-name soul foods in their listings of brand-name foods.

To that end, the objectives of this book are:

- To help African Americans with diabetes understand how soul food will impact blood glucose levels and self-management of diabetes

- To facilitate the intake of healthful foods and planning of healthy meals

- To shorten the cultural distance between patients and diabetes educators

- To increase patient satisfaction

This comprehensive guide is written for African Americans with diabetes, their families, diabetes educators, dietetic professionals, and anyone with diabetes who eats traditional foods from the South and the Caribbean.

To prepare the brand-name convenience soul food nutrient information, food companies were contacted to obtain current nutrition information for their products. Exchanges and carbohydrate choices were calculated based on this information.

Sources for Caribbean food nutrition data:

Food Composition Tables: Caribbean Food and Nutrition Institute, second edition revised.
Pan American Health Organization
Kingston, Jamaica, 1998

Food Composition: Caribbean Food and Nutrition Institute, supplement.
Pan American Health Organization
Kingston, Jamaica, 2000

Sources for soul food, Cajun, and Creole food nutrition data:

Diet Analysis+, Version 6.0
ESHA Research, Wadsworth (a division of Thomson Learning Company)
2003

Food: A Handbook of Terminology, Purchasing, and Preparation, tenth edition
American Association of Family and Consumer Sciences
Alexandria, VA, 2001

Exchange Lists for Meal Planning
American Dietetic Association, American Diabetes Association
2003

Nutritive Values of Foods
USDA Home and Garden Bulletin 72
2002

Acknowledgments

Many thanks to my husband Lawrence and our family and friends for all their encouragement and support.

Special thanks to the following people for their time and talent:

Susan Kelly, graphic artist—cover design

Sana Khan, graphic artist—interior illustrations.

JoAnn Randazzo, RD—compilation of nutrient data

Jeffery Howard Shiff, MD, Endocrinologist, who took time out of his busy schedule to review this book and provide his invaluable editing suggestions.

Karen Notgarnie, CPVA, for her keen eye, editorial review and administrative assistance.

List of Abbreviations

c	cup
cal	calorie
carb	carbohydrate
CHO	carbohydrate exchange
choc	chocolate
conc	concentrate
dL	deciliter (1/10 of a liter)
fl	fluid ounce
frzn	frozen
g	gram
lo-cal	low-calorie
mg	milligram
med	medium
NA	not available
ND	not determined
oz	ounce
pcs	pieces
pkg	package
RDA	Recommended Dietary Allowance

sat	saturated
sm	small
sod	sodium
sq	square
swtned	sweetened
tbsp	tablespoon
tr	trace
tsp	teaspoon
μg	microgram
vit	vitamin
w/	with

Part I

The Diabetes Epidemic in African Americans: Stating the Case

Chapter 1

A Little Sugar

A little sugar, a touch of sugar, sugar in the blood, or sugar diabetes…some people think "a touch a sugar" is a mild form of diabetes. But who's kidding who? You either have diabetes, or you don't. There is no such thing as "a little sugar," and diabetes is not caused by eating too much sugar.

Diabetes is a disease that causes your blood glucose (blood sugar) levels to remain above normal. People with diabetes have trouble converting food to energy. After eating—especially foods containing carbohydrates, like bread, cereal, fruit, vegetable and milk—the pancreas is alerted to make a hormone called insulin. The job of insulin is to take glucose out of the bloodstream and help it to enter the cells of the body, where the glucose can be stored or used as a source of energy. When you have diabetes, this process does not happen as it should. Either your body does not make enough insulin or insulin is not used properly. The end result is a buildup of glucose in your blood that, over the years, can have serious health consequences. Too much glucose in the blood can damage nerves and blood vessels, which can ultimately result in heart disease, stroke, blindness, kidney disease, nerve problems, gum infections, and amputations.

There are three main kinds of diabetes: type 1 diabetes, type 2 diabetes, and gestational diabetes.

Type 1 Diabetes

When you have type 1 diabetes, your body is not able to make enough of its own insulin to keep your blood sugar levels normal. People with type 1 diabetes require daily insulin injections to live. Because of this, type 1 diabetes was previously called insulin-dependent diabetes mellitus (IDDM) or juvenile-onset diabetes, because it usually occurred in childhood or adolescence.

However, it may occur at any age. Approximately 1 out of every 10 people with diabetes has type 1.

Type 2 Diabetes

In type 2 diabetes, your body either does not make enough insulin (which is called insulin deficiency), or the cells in the muscles, liver, and fat do not use insulin properly (which is called insulin resistance).

Type 2 diabetes is the most common type of diabetes. 9 out of every 10 people diagnosed with diabetes have type 2. Type 2 diabetes, once thought of as an adult disease, has now reached epidemic proportions among our youth (see Chapter 3).

Type 2 diabetes most often occurs in people who:

- Are over 40 years of age
- Are overweight or physically inactive
- Have a family history of diabetes
- Have a history of diabetes during pregnancy (gestational diabetes)
- Have given birth to a large baby weighing over 9 pounds
- Are African American, Hispanic/Latino American or American Indian

Gestational Diabetes

Some women develop gestational diabetes during the late stages of pregnancy. Gestational diabetes is caused by the hormones of pregnancy or a shortage of insulin. Gestational diabetes occurs most frequently among African American, Hispanic/Latino Americans, and American Indians. It is most common among obese women and women with a family history of diabetes. Although this form of diabetes usually goes away after the baby is born, a woman who has had gestational diabetes has a 20% to 50% chance of developing diabetes in the next 5 to 10 years, and is more likely to develop type 2 diabetes later in life.

Managing your Diabetes

When you have diabetes, you are asked to make a number of changes in your behavior and lifestyle. You will be much more successful in making these changes if you have a clear understanding of what is going on inside your body. Insulin deficiency and insulin resistance are the two main problems in type 2 diabetes.

Insulin is often thought of as the key that unlocks the doors of the cells in your body, allowing glucose to enter the cells, where it can be used for energy. Glucose is the body's main source of fuel, much like gasoline is your car's main source of fuel. Simply put, insulin deficiency is like driving a Cadillac with a Volkswagen engine.

In insulin resistance, the cells in the muscles, liver, and fat do not use insulin properly. It's as if the cell doors no longer recognize insulin and won't open to allow glucose in. Another explanation is to think of the cell as being hard-of-hearing and that insulin is knocking at the cell door.

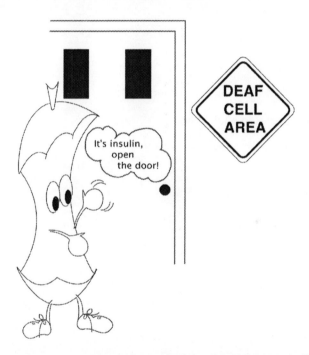

As insulin continues to knock at the cell door, the amount of glucose in the blood increases, while the cells are starved of energy. The lack of energy triggers a chain reaction. The cell sends a signal to the brain that it needs energy. The brain then sends a signal to the pancreas to release more insulin to knock at the cell door and get glucose into the cell for energy. Eventually, the cell will hear insulin knocking and open the door, allowing glucose in. Over time, the pancreas becomes "tired" and is no longer able to produce the additional insulin necessary to get glucose into the cell. Blood insulin levels finally fall, causing further increases in blood glucose levels.

Both insulin deficiency and insulin resistance cause your blood glucose levels to remain higher than normal. Symptoms of high blood glucose include the following:

- Increased thirst

- Extreme hunger

- Frequent urination

- Feeling tired

- Itchy or dry skin

- Slow-healing cuts or sores

- More infections than usual

- Tingling or numbness in hands or feet

- Unexplained weight loss

- Sudden vision changes

Chapter 2

Is Diabetes Different in African Americans?

African Americans have the same risk factors for diabetes as other popula-
tions. However, African Americans are unique in terms of the outcomes of diabetes complications, which are much more devastating in African Americans.
For every 6 white Americans who have diabetes, 10 African Americans have
the disease.

An estimated 2.8 million African Americans 20 years or older have diabetes;
1.5 million have been diagnosed, and 730,000 don't know they have the disease. There are 4 times as many African Americans diagnosed with diabetes
today than in 1968. According to the Centers for Disease Control, in 2002,
diabetes was the fourth leading cause of death in African Americans. African
Americans with diabetes are more likely to develop diabetes complications
and experience greater disability from the complications than white Americans
with diabetes.

Heart disease is the leading cause of diabetes-related deaths. Adults with
diabetes have heart-disease-related death rates about 2 to 4 times higher than
adults without diabetes. The risk for stroke is also 2 to 4 times higher among
people with diabetes.

Diabetic retinopathy, disorders of the retina, causes 12,000 to 24,000 new
cases of blindness each year. Diabetes is the leading cause of new cases of
blindness among adults aged 20 to 74 years. African Americans are twice as
likely to suffer from diabetes-related blindness.

Diabetes kidney disease (also called diabetic nephropathy)—Diabetes is the leading cause of end-stage renal disease (also called kidney failure), accounting for 44% of new cases. According to the National Institute of Diabetes & Digestive & Kidney Diseases (NIDDK) in 2001, a total of 142,963 people with end-stage renal disease due to diabetes were living on dialysis or with a kidney transplant. African Americans with diabetes experience kidney failure about four times more often than diabetic white Americans.

Amputations—More than 60% of nontraumatic lower limb amputations in the U.S. occur among people with diabetes. Each year 82,000 people lose their foot or leg to diabetes. African Americans are much more likely to undergo a lower limb amputation than white or Hispanic Americans with diabetes.

While the statistics sound devastating, the good news is that there are steps you can take to prevent these diabetes complications:

- Keep blood sugar levels under control.

- Maintain a healthy weight.

- Eat the right amounts of a variety of foods.

- Get regular physical activity.

- Take diabetes medicine as prescribed.

- Monitor blood sugar levels.

In Part II, "Fighting the Diabetes Epidemic," you will learn how to mount an effective defense against the complications of diabetes.

Chapter 3

Diabetes and Our Children

Type 2 diabetes, as discussed in Chapter 1, is a disease commonly found in obese adults. However, recent statistics indicate that type 2 diabetes is now emerging rapidly as an epidemic in our children and adolescents. Why is this happening? Well, this rise is a direct result of the epidemic of obesity that has hit our nation with a vengeance. Obesity has not only risen in adults, but over the past two decades, the rate of obesity has doubled in children.

Obesity causes insulin resitance and is therefore a major risk factor for type 2 diabetes. In insulin resistance, the body may be producing enough insulin, but it is unable to use the insulin properly. Research shows that the greater the degree of obesity in our children, the greater the degree of not only insulin resistance, but high blood pressure and high triglyceride levels. This can ultimately lead to diabetes, stroke, and heart disease.

With these alarming facts in mind, you might want to think twice when you laugh about those *pudgy cheeks and ham-hock legs on your little dumpling*. As a matter of fact, ask yourself, is this cute? Or is it the picture of a disease waiting to happen? Don't forget, if you have type 2 diabetes, then whoever your little dumpling is—a child, grandchild, niece, or nephew—he or she might be at risk as well.

A common sign of insulin resistance is acanthosis (uh-kan-THO-sis) nigricans (NIH-grih-kans), which is a skin condition often seen in obese individuals predisposed to develop pre-diabetes and type 2 diabetes. Acanthosis nigricans causes darkened skin patches on the neck and armpits. There is no doubt that you have previously observed this skin condition on someone you know. You might have mistaken it for a dirty neck.

Your Child's Risk for Type 2 Diabetes

Your child is at risk if he or she is…

- African American
- Overweight
- Inactive
- Insulin resistant
- Going through puberty
- Born small or large

And especially if he or she is

- Born into a family has with a history of type 2 diabetes

In addition to the risk factors for type 2 diabetes in children, there are warning signs. Children should be observed for increased thirst, frequent urination, blurry vision, nighttime urination, unexplained weight loss, fatigue—and don't forget that dark skin around the neck.

Can type 2 diabetes be prevented?

Studies have shown that weight management, healthy food choices—including low-fat, high-fiber foods—and increased physical activity can delay or prevent the onset of type 2 diabetes. For many, however, this may mean a total lifestyle change. Parents must start evaluating how they feed their children, what they feed them, how much they feed them, and certainly how much exercise the children are getting. As in every aspect of raising children, the parent is the best example. If you overeat, your children will overeat. The good news is that when exposed to positive role models, children can learn to make healthy food choices.

Not sure where to begin?

Start with the "Healthful Eating and Lifestyle Tips" noted in the following table. Remember, these are general guidelines. Don't expect to make all the changes at once. Research shows that you will be more successful with small, gradual changes over time. For a complete assessment and evaluation, consult a registered dietitian (RD) in your area. An RD is a nutrition expert who can assist with meal planning and menu makeovers.

Healthful Eating and Lifestyle Tips

- Limit television and video games to less than 4 hours a day.

- Encourage an after-school sports activity.

- Plan family activities that require movement, such as skating, swimming, or basketball.

- Limit portion sizes.

- Offer low-fat snacks, such as popcorn, low-fat crackers, and pretzels.

- Offer low-fat milk and milk products.

- Offer more water instead of regular soda, sport drinks, and fruit drinks.

- Limit fast foods and pizza to once or twice a week.

- Serve fewer fried and high-fat starches, such as regular biscuits, corn bread, pancakes, or waffles.

- Buy whole-grain breads, cereal, rice, and pasta.

- Offer fresh fruit instead of sugary canned fruit.

- Steam vegetables using a small amount of water or low-fat broth; add a small piece of lean ham or smoked turkey if desired.

Chapter 4

Hope for the Future

If you have diabetes, there is a good chance that someone you love is at risk for developing diabetes as well.

The results of a major study called the Diabetes Prevention Program (DPP) provide hope for your loved ones and other people at risk of developing type 2 diabetes. This study involved 3,234 people, half of whom were African American, American Indian, Asian American, Pacific Islander, or Hispanic/Latino American. Participants were overweight and had higher-than-normal blood glucose, a condition called pre-diabetes. If your blood glucose is higher than normal, but lower than the diabetes range, you have pre-diabetes. Both pre-diabetes and obesity are risk factors for type 2 diabetes.

The DPP tested two approaches to preventing the progression from pre-diabetes to diabetes: lifestyle modification involving healthy eating and exercise, and a second approach using the diabetes drug metformin (Glucophage). People in the lifestyle modification group walked about 30 minutes a day, 5 days a week, and lowered their intake of fat and calories. Those who took the diabetes drug metformin (Glucophage) received standard information on exercise and diet. The results showed that people in the lifestyle modification group reduced their risk of getting type 2 diabetes by 58%. Additionally, they lost an average of 15 pounds. Lifestyle modification was even more effective in those 60 and older; they reduced their risk by 71%.

If you weigh more than your ideal weight and have a family history of diabetes, you should discuss testing for pre-diabetes with your health-care provider during a regular check-up.

If you or someone you love is at risk of developing type 2 diabetes, there are steps you can take to lower that risk. Remember, there is no cure for diabetes, but prevention is possible.

Steps to Lower the Risk of Getting Diabetes:

- Reach and maintain a reasonable body weight (see chapter 6).

- Make wise food choices most of the time (see chapter 7).

- Be physically active every day (see chapter 8).

Part II

Fighting the Diabetes Epidemic in African Americans: Mounting Your Defense

Chapter 5

Become an Educated Consumer

In 1922, Dr. Elliott Joslin, founder of the Joslin Diabetes Center and credited with developing the concept of the "diabetes team," said, "The patient, who knows the most, lives the longest." Since that time, research shows that knowing does not always translate into doing. However, knowledge is power, and knowledge can help you successfully manage diabetes. With diabetes education and behavior changes, you can reduce the risk of complications such as heart disease, kidney disease, amputation, and blindness.

This book is a good starting point in becoming an educated consumer and learning about diabetes. Many hospitals and clinics have diabetes education programs where they will teach you important skills, like monitoring your blood sugar, planning your meals, taking your medications, and using insulin.

Teaming up with a Certified Diabetes Educator (CDE) is another way to become knowledgeable about diabetes. Diabetes educators are health professionals, primarily nurses, dietitians, and pharmacists, who specialize in providing care and education to people with diabetes. Doctors, exercise physiologists, podiatrists, and social workers may also specialize in diabetes education and may hold the CDE credential. Diabetes is a complicated disease that requires a multidisciplinary team for effective management. Diabetes educators work in a variety of settings, such as hospitals, doctors' offices, nursing homes, and clinics.

Diabetes Dream Team

- Primary care physician

- Endocrinologist—diabetes specialist

- Certified Diabetes Educator—nurse and/or registered dietitian

- Ophthalmologist—eye doctor

- Podiatrist—foot doctor

- Pharmacist

A diagnosis of diabetes can be met with many feelings, such as fear, shock, guilt, denial, depression, and even blame. These are all normal feelings. Your attitudes, beliefs, and values will also play a role in your response to living with a life-long disease. Many attitudes and beliefs about diabetes are based on misinformation and anecdotes given by family and friends. A diabetes educator will work with you to examine your feelings and fears about living with diabetes. By getting to know you on an individual basis, a diabetes educator will help create a self-management plan that meets your needs, based on your age, school or work schedule, family demands, eating habits, and health problems.

Diabetes Educators Help You

- Understand the disease process

- Make healthy food choices

- Develop a fitness plan

- Understand how your medication works

- Understand when and how to take your medication

- Learn how to monitor your blood sugar

- Reflect on your attitudes, beliefs and values

- Accept the realities of diabetes

- Learn how to problem-solve

Diabetes treatment and management is constantly changing, therefore you must keep learning as much as you can. Subscribe to diabetes-related magazines, such as The American Diabetes Association's *Diabetes Forecast.* Go to the American Diabetes Association's Web site, www.diabetes.org, to read the latest in diabetes research and treatment advances. Your local Diabetes Association can help you find an approved Diabetes Education Program in your area or a diabetes support group.

To locate a diabetes educator near you, go to the American Association of Diabetes Educators Web site at www.aadenet.org and choose "Diabetes Education;" then choose "Find a Diabetes Educator." Or call 1-800-832-6874.

Chapter 6

Shed Those Pounds

More than 80% of people with type 2 diabetes are overweight. If you have diabetes and are overweight, it is likely that you have insulin resistance as well. Being overweight changes the way the cells in the body respond to insulin, as illustrated in Chapter 1 with the deaf cell. Additionally, in time, your pancreas will begin to make less insulin. Remember, if you are overweight and your pancreas is not making enough insulin, it is similar to driving a Cadillac with a Volkswagen engine. In other words, your pancreas just can't keep up with the demands of your body.

Losing as little as between 10 and 15 pounds will improve the cells' response to insulin and help control your blood sugar levels: you'll trade that Cadillac in for a brand-new Volkswagen! Weight loss may also reduce the amount of diabetes medication you take, improve blood cholesterol and triglyceride levels, and improve your blood pressure.

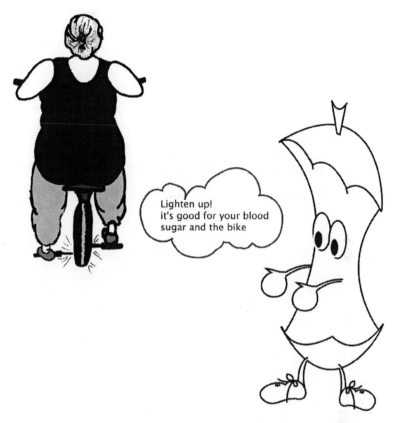

There are two common reasons for being overweight: eating too much and not being active enough. If you eat more calories than your body burns up, the extra calories are stored as fat. We all need a little stored fat to serve as a cushion for the body's frame and to protect our organs. But too much fat results in being overweight. Where your fat is located can also cause more problems. If your fat is located in the abdominal area, or you are shaped like an apple, you are at greater risk for heart disease. If you are shaped like a pear and your fat is located in the hips and thighs, your risk for heart disease is less. Waist measurements more than 40 inches for men and 35 inches for women are indicators of increased risk for heart disease and high blood pressure.

Body Mass Index (BMI) is another measurement that helps to assess your weight and risk for disease and death. BMI is a measure of your weight in relation to your height and is used as an estimate of your body fat. Combining the BMI and waist measurement will tell you your risk for developing other obesity-associated disease.

What Is Your Risk?

Follow the steps outlined below to find out your obesity-related disease risk.

1. Use the BMI tables on pages 25 and 26 to estimate your total body fat. Locate your height in the left-hand column and read across the row for that height to your body weight. Follow the column of your weight up to the top row that lists the BMI. The BMI scores mean the following:

Below 18.5	Underweight
18.5–24.9	Normal
25.0–29.9	Overweight
30.0 and above	Obese

2. Measure your waist by placing a measuring tape snugly around your waist where your belly button is.

3. Now, with your BMI and waist size determined, use the following table to determine your health risk relative to normal weight.

Risk of Associated Disease According to BMI and Waist Size			
BMI		Waist less than or equal to 40 in. (men) or 35 in. (women)	Waist greater than 40 in. (men) or 35 in. (women)
18.5 or less	Underweight		N/A
18.5–24.9	Normal		N/A
25.0–29.9	Overweight	Increased	High
30.0–34.9	Obese	High	Very High
35.0–39.9	Obese	Very High	Very High
40 or greater	Extremely Obese	Extremely High	Extremely High

From: http://www.nhlbi.nih.gov/healthpublic/heart/obesity/lose_wt/bmi_dis.htm

You should lose weight if you are…

- Obese (BMI greater than or equal to 30)

- Overweight (BMI of 25 to 29.9) and have two or more of the following risk factors:
    - High blood pressure (hypertension)
    - High LDL-cholesterol ("bad" cholesterol)
    - Low HDL-cholesterol ("good" cholesterol)
    - High triglycerides
    - High blood glucose (sugar)
    - Family history of premature heart disease
    - Physical inactivity
    - Cigarette smoking

If you need to lose weight, a slow, gradual weight loss of 1/2–1 lb weekly is recommended. For moderate weight loss, women should aim for about 1,200 calories daily. Men should aim for 1,400 daily. Use the chart below to determine your daily calorie needs based on your current weight.

<u>Daily Calorie Requirement</u>

Current weight × 10 for weight loss

Current weight × 12 for weight maintenance

Current weight × 15 for weight gain

The table below is based on the exchange system for meal planning. It can be used as a guide in your daily meal planning. It provides you with the right number of daily servings from each food group, based on your calorie needs. In the exchange system, foods are categorized based on the amount of carbohydrates, protein, and fat they contain. Each group lists food in serving sizes. You can exchange, trade, or substitute a food serving in the same group. In Part IV you will find the exchange values for many of your favorite foods. To achieve your weight goals, choose a calorie level that is close to your daily calorie requirement. Follow the column of your calorie level down to determine the appropriate number of daily servings from each food group. In Chapter 7, will learn what a serving size is and how to make healthy food choices.

Sample Meal Patterns

Daily servings from each food group	1200 calorie	1500 calorie	1800 calorie	2000 calorie	2500 calorie
Starch	5	7	8	9	11
Fruit	3	3	4	4	6
Milk	2	2	3	3	3
Vegetables	2	2	3	3	5
Meat/Meat Substitutes	4	4	6	6	8
Fat	3	4	4	5	6

To get more help losing weight and to individualize your meal plan, see a Registered Dietitian (RD). You can locate an RD in your area by calling the American Dietetic Association at 800-877-1600, or log on to www.eatright.org and click on "Find a Nutrition Professional."

BMI	19	20	21	22	23	24	25	26	27	28	29	30	31	32	33	34	35
Height (inches)	Body Weight (pounds)																
58	91	96	100	105	110	115	119	124	129	134	138	143	148	153	158	162	167
59	94	99	104	109	114	119	124	128	133	138	143	148	153	158	163	168	173
60	97	102	107	112	118	123	128	133	138	143	148	153	158	163	168	174	179
61	100	106	111	116	122	127	132	137	143	148	153	158	164	169	174	180	185
62	104	109	115	120	126	131	136	142	147	153	158	164	169	175	180	186	191
63	107	113	118	124	130	135	141	146	152	158	163	169	175	180	186	191	197
64	110	116	122	128	134	140	145	151	157	163	169	174	180	186	192	197	204
65	114	120	126	132	138	144	150	156	162	168	174	180	186	192	198	204	210
66	118	124	130	136	142	148	155	161	167	173	179	186	192	198	204	210	216
67	121	127	134	140	146	153	159	166	172	178	185	191	198	204	211	217	223
68	125	131	138	144	151	158	164	171	177	184	190	197	203	210	216	223	230
69	128	135	142	149	155	162	169	176	182	189	196	203	209	216	223	230	236
70	132	139	146	153	160	167	174	181	188	195	202	209	216	222	229	236	243
71	136	143	150	157	165	172	179	186	193	200	208	215	222	229	236	243	250
72	140	147	154	162	169	177	184	191	199	206	213	221	228	235	242	250	258
73	144	151	159	166	174	182	189	197	204	212	219	227	235	242	250	257	265
74	148	155	163	171	179	186	194	202	210	218	225	233	241	249	256	264	272
75	152	160	168	176	184	192	200	208	216	224	232	240	248	256	264	272	279
76	156	164	172	180	189	197	205	213	221	230	238	246	254	263	271	279	287

BMI	36	37	38	39	40	41	42	43	44	45	46	47	48	49	50	51	52	53	54
Height (inches)	Body Weight (pounds)																		
58	172	177	181	186	191	196	201	205	210	215	220	224	229	234	239	244	248	253	258
59	178	183	188	193	198	203	208	212	217	222	227	232	237	242	247	252	257	262	267
60	184	189	194	199	204	209	215	220	225	230	235	240	245	250	255	261	266	271	276
61	190	195	201	206	211	217	222	227	232	238	243	248	254	259	264	269	275	280	285
62	196	202	207	213	218	224	229	235	240	246	251	256	262	267	273	278	284	289	295
63	203	208	214	220	225	231	237	242	248	254	259	265	270	278	282	287	293	299	304
64	209	215	221	227	232	238	244	250	256	262	267	273	279	285	291	296	302	308	314
65	216	222	228	234	240	246	252	258	264	270	276	282	288	294	300	306	312	318	324
66	223	229	235	241	247	253	260	266	272	278	284	291	297	303	309	315	322	328	334
67	230	236	242	249	255	261	268	274	280	287	293	299	306	312	319	325	331	338	344
68	236	243	249	256	262	269	276	282	289	295	302	308	315	322	328	335	341	348	354
69	243	250	257	263	270	277	284	291	297	304	311	318	324	331	338	345	351	358	365
70	250	257	264	271	278	285	292	299	306	313	320	327	334	341	348	355	362	369	376
71	257	265	272	279	286	293	301	308	315	322	329	338	343	351	358	365	372	379	386
72	265	272	279	287	294	302	309	316	324	331	338	346	353	361	368	375	383	390	397
73	272	280	288	295	302	310	318	325	333	340	348	355	363	371	378	386	393	401	408
74	280	287	295	303	311	319	326	334	342	350	358	365	373	381	389	396	404	412	420
75	287	295	303	311	319	327	335	343	351	359	367	375	383	391	399	407	415	423	431
76	295	304	312	320	328	336	344	353	361	369	377	385	394	402	410	418	426	435	443

From: http://www.nhlbisupport.com/bmi/bmicalc.htm

Chapter 7

Improve Food Choices

Now that you've done the math and figured out your calorie needs, the next step is to figure out what you should eat. Weight loss does not mean starvation or following some fad diet. It's also important to remember that you can't starve yourself to get control of your blood glucose levels. However, you might have to rethink some of your current eating behaviors and improve your food choices.

The principles of healthy eating for the person with diabetes are the same as for the general population. And if you eat traditional Soul, Caribbean, or Creole food, you'll be happy to know that many traditional dishes like beans, peas, lentils, and dark green vegetables such as collard greens, cabbage, spinach, and turnip greens can be eaten as well. They are high in fiber, vitamins, and minerals and low in fat. Sweet potatoes and corn bread are also good sources of fiber. Yes, it may require eating a little less of this and more of that. But the bottom line is everyone needs a variety of food on a daily basis to get all the nutrients the body needs for good health. The food you eat should provide enough carbohydrates, protein, fat, vitamins, minerals, fiber, and water. All of these nutrients working together give you the energy you need for a full and productive lifestyle.

Carbohydrates are your body's preferred source of energy and should make up 45% to 60% of your daily calories. Carbohydrates provide 4 calories per gram. Contrary to what many of the popular fad diets tell us, your body needs carbohydrates, and carbohydrates are part of a healthful diet. Now, you're probably saying, "I thought carbohydrates were bad for people with diabetes." No, carbohydrates are not bad, but if you eat too much of them at a meal or snack, they will cause your blood glucose level to go up. In Chapter 11, "The

Choice Is Yours," you will learn how you can successfully make carbohydrates part of your daily meal plan.

The three main types of carbohydrates are sugar, starch, and fiber.

Sugar is sometimes called simple sugar or fast-acting carbohydrate. Table sugar, cane sugar, brown sugar, maple syrup, molasses, honey, turbinado sugar, and high-fructose corn syrup are all sugars. Fruit sugar (fructose) and milk sugar (lactose) are also sugars. Foods made with sugar tend to have little or no nutritional value, and are usually high in calories and fat. The sugar in fruit and milk is naturally occurring and comes with many nutrients, like the fiber in fruit and the calcium in milk.

Starch is the second type of carbohydrate. Starch is made from sugars that are linked together in long chains. Foods high in starch include bread, cereal, pasta, crackers, and starchy vegetables (peas, corn, lima beans, and potatoes), dried beans, lentils, and peas (such as pinto beans, kidney beans, black-eyed peas, and split peas). During digestion, all simple sugars and starches are converted to glucose and therefore affect your blood glucose level more than any other nutrient.

Fiber is the third type of carbohydrate. Fiber is the indigestible part of plant food. It includes the leaves of vegetables, fruit skins, and seeds. Fiber slows the digestion of starches to glucose, keeping the blood sugar more stable. Because fiber can't be digested completely, it adds bulk and helps to move food waste out of the body more quickly. Some good sources of fiber are as follows:

- Whole-grain products, including breads from whole wheat, rye, bran, oat, and corn flour or cornmeal, pastas; whole-grain or bran cereals; brown rice

- Vegetables, such as broccoli, Brussels sprouts, cabbage, carrots, green beans and peas, lentils, dried beans and peas, sweet potatoes, turnips, and all forms of greens, cooked or raw, and other vegetables

- Fruits, such as apples, bananas, berries, cantaloupes, kiwi, oranges, peaches, grapes, pears, watermelon and other melons, and dried fruits, such as raisins and dried apricots

- Nuts and seeds

Nutrition Guidelines for Carbohydrates and Diabetes

- Food containing carbohydrates from whole grains, fruits, vegetables, and low-fat milk should be included in a healthy diet.

- The total amount of carbohydrates in meals and snacks is more important than the source or type.

- Sugar can be substituted for other carbohydrate sources in a meal.

- 45% to 60% of total calories should come from carbohydrates.

- A healthy fiber intake is 20–35 grams daily or 14 grams per 1000 calories.

Protein

Like carbohydrates, protein provides energy for the body; however, it is not the preferred energy source. Protein provides 4 calories per gram. Protein is made up of building blocks called amino acids that can be found in both plant and animal sources. There are 20 different amino acids. Of these 20 amino acids, 9 are considered essential, because the body cannot make them on its own. Essential amino acids must come from the food you eat.

Protein can be found in every cell of the body. Your organs, muscles, nervous system, blood vessels, and skeleton are all dependent on protein. It is used to build and repair body tissue and keep your hair, fingernails, and skin healthy. Protein also helps to boost your immune system.

Protein is found in both plant and animal sources. Protein from animals contains all of the essential amino acids and is therefore called a "complete" protein. Meat, fish, dairy, and eggs are good sources of complete proteins. Plant protein does not contain enough of one or more of the essential amino acids. Grains, legumes, nuts, and seeds are good sources of plant proteins. Eating a large variety of plant protein will help you get all of the essential amino acids.

Soy foods are the exception to the rule. Soy foods are the only plant-based foods that contain all nine essential amino acids. Soy is the only plant food that is a "complete" protein.

Nutrition Guidelines for Protein and Diabetes

- 15%–20% of total calories should come from protein.

- Choose protein sources that are low in saturated fat and cholesterol, such as poultry, fish, legumes, beans (soy, pinto, black, kidney), grains, nuts, low fat dairy and egg whites.

- It is not necessary to have a protein source at each meal.

- If you have well controlled type 2 diabetes, protein will not cause a rise in your blood glucose levels.

Fat and Cholesterol

Fat is the most concentrated source of energy for the body, providing 9 calories per gram, more than double the amount found in carbohydrates and protein. Energy is stored in the body mostly in the form of fat, and fat is essential to insulate the body tissues, protect the vital organs, and transport and absorb the fat-soluble vitamins A, D, E, and K. Fat also plays a very important role in food flavor and texture. Fat enhances food flavor, provides a smooth, silky mouth-feel, makes baked products tender, and helps prevent sticking.

Fats are made up of fatty acids that are linked together. There are three types of fatty acids: saturated, monounsaturated, and polyunsaturated. All fats and oils are made up of a combination of these three fatty acids. The predominate type of fat in a food determines which category the food falls into.

Saturated fatty acids are usually solid at room temperature and are found mostly in foods coming from animals, such as meat, lard, bacon, poultry, dairy products, butterfat, and eggs. Oils such as coconut, palm kernel oil, and palm oil fall into the category of saturated fats. Saturated fat can cause your body to produce too much cholesterol.

Monounsaturated fatty acids are usually liquid at room temperature and are found mostly in vegetable oils such as canola, olive, and peanut oils, and whole olives and peanuts. Monounsaturated fats are often called heart-healthy fats, because they do not cause your cholesterol level to rise. However, it is important to remember that when it comes to calories, "fat is fat," and all types provide 9 calories per gram.

Polyunsaturated fatty acids are usually liquid or soft at room temperature and are found mostly in vegetable oils, such as safflower, sunflower, corn, flaxseed, and canola oils. Fatty fish such as salmon, albacore tuna, herring, and mackerel also contain a type of polyunsaturated fat called omega-3 fatty acids, which are thought to be helpful in lowering triglyceride levels. Walnuts are also a good source of omega-3 fatty acids. Just as there are essential amino acids, there are essential fatty acids needed by the body for cell structure and hormone formation. Linoleic acid and alpha-linolenic acid are the two essential polyunsaturated fatty acids and must be obtained from the foods we eat. Linoleic acid is found in vegetable oils—soybean, corn, and safflower are good sources. Alpha-linolenic acid is found mostly in fatty fish such as albacore, mackerel, salmon and tuna.

Trans-fatty acids are a relatively new category that has been added. These are polyunsaturated fats that have been chemically changed to make them solid at room temperature. Hydrogenated vegetable oils, such as vegetable shortening and margarine, contain trans-fatty acids. There is evidence these fatty acids may be harmful to cholesterol profiles.

Cholesterol is a waxy substance found in the blood that occurs naturally in your body. All the cholesterol the body needs is made by the liver. Cholesterol is also found in foods of animal origin, such as egg yolks, organ meats like liver, and full-fat dairy products like milk, cheese, and meat. Cholesterol is used to build cell membranes and brain and nerve tissues. It also helps the body form hormones needed for body regulation, including processing food, and bile acids needed for digestion.

Cholesterol is carried in the bloodstream in packages of fat and protein called lipoproteins. Cholesterol carried in packages called low density lipoproteins is called LDL cholesterol or "bad" cholesterol. Cholesterol carried in packages called high density lipoproteins is called HDL cholesterol or "good" cholesterol.

LDL cholesterol and HDL cholesterol act differently in the body. A high level of LDL cholesterol can increase the risk of heart disease, because it causes fatty deposits to form in the arteries. A high level of HDL cholesterol seems to have a protective effect against heart disease, because it helps to remove excess cholesterol from the blood and carry it to the liver, where it can be excreted.

Cholesterol and Fat Goals

HDL cholesterol	over 40 **mg/dL for men
	over 50 mg/dL for women
LDL cholesterol	under 100 mg/dL
	under 70 mg/dL for high-risk individuals
*Triglycerides	under 150 mg/dL
Total cholesterol	under 200 mg/dL

*Triglycerides are the storage form of fat.
**mg/dL—a volume measure of blood

Nutrition Guidelines for Fat and Cholesterol and Diabetes

- Limit total daily calories from fat to 20–30%.

- Limit total daily calories from saturated fat to 7–10 %.

- Consume less than 300 mg cholesterol daily.

- Choose low fat and reduced calorie foods wisely because they can contain more carbohydrate than the full fat food.

- Consume 3–4 servings of fish weekly.

- Avoid organ meats like liver.

Vitamins and Minerals

Vitamins are needed for normal growth and development of the body. Vitamins do not provide energy, but they do help the body break down carbohydrates, protein, and fat and use them more efficiently. The body requires very small quantities of vitamins, but it cannot function properly without them.

Vitamins fit into two basic classifications: water-soluble and fat-soluble.

Water-soluble vitamins cannot be stored and must be taken into the body on a daily basis. The water-soluble vitamins are B and C.

Fat-soluble vitamins A, D, E, and K are stored in the liver and fat tissue of the body. Fat-soluble vitamins can be toxic to the body if taken in large quantities. (See chart "Daily Vitamin and Mineral Guide")

There is no clear evidence that people with diabetes who do not have vitamin or mineral deficiencies will benefit from supplementation. However, if you plan to use a vitamin or mineral supplement, make sure you discuss it with your doctor or health-care provider. Many supplements contain active ingredients that have strong biological effects, and their safety is not always assured in all users. Other supplements may interact with prescription and over-the-counter medicines. By taking these products, you may be placing yourself at risk.

Daily Vitamin and Mineral Guide

	Function	Food Source	Recommended Dietary Allowance	Tolerable upper intake level/adverse effects
Vitamin A	Normal vision, growth, development, and reproduction. Healthy skin, teeth, and bones. Also helps fight infection	Liver, dairy products, fish, darkly colored fruits and leafy vegetables	700 µg/day for women 900 µg/day for men	3,000 µg/day Liver toxicity
Vitamin B_6	Normal growth. Also participates in enzyme systems for metabolism of protein and carbohydrates	Fortified cereals, organ meats, fortified soy-based meat substitutes	1.3 mg/day	100 mg/day Sensory neuropathy (nerve damage)
Vitamin B_{12}	Keeps red blood cells and the nervous system healthy; participates in energy metabolism	Fortified cereals, meat, fish, poultry	2.4 µg/day	Not determined

	Function	Food Source	Recommended Dietary Allowance	Tolerable upper intake level/adverse effects
Folic Acid	Prevents birth defects. Participates in formation of red blood cells, metabolism of protein, and normal digestive system functions	Enriched cereal grains, dark leafy vegetables, enriched and whole-grain breads and bread products, fortified ready-to-eat cereals	400 µg/day	1,000 µg/day Upper limit applies to synthetic forms obtained from supplements and/or fortified foods
Niacin	Helps release energy, promotes good physical and mental health, healthy skin, tongue, and digestive system	Meat, fish, poultry, enriched and whole-grain breads and bread products, fortified ready-to-eat cereals	14 mg/day for women 16 mg/day for men	35 mg/day Upper limit applies to synthetic forms obtained from supplements and/or fortified foods High levels associated with flushing (redness of the skin)
Riboflavin	Helps release energy. Promotes growth and cellular metabolism, healthy eyes, skin, lips, and tongue	Organ meats, milk, bread products, and fortified cereals	1.1 mg/day for women 1.3 mg/day for men	Not determined

	Function	Food Source	Recommended Dietary Allowance	Tolerable upper intake level/adverse effects
Thiamin	Participates in the metabolism of carbohydrates and protein.	Enriched, fortified, or whole-grain products, bread and bread products, mixed foods whose main ingredient is grain, and ready-to-eat cereals	1.1 mg/day for women 1.3 mg/day for men	Not determined
Vitamin C	Helps maintain body tissue and promote wound healing. Protects the body against infection and oxidative destruction	Citrus fruits, tomatoes, tomato juice, potatoes, Brussels sprouts, cauliflower, broccoli, strawberries, cabbage, and spinach	75 mg/day for women 90 mg/day for men	2,000 mg/day Diarrhea and other gastrointestinal disturbances
Vitamin E	Prevents oxidative destruction of cell membranes	Vegetable oils, unprocessed cereal grains, nuts, fruits, vegetables, meats	15 mg/day as α-tocopherol	1,000 mg/day Hemorrhage

	Function	Food Source	Recommended Dietary Allowance	Tolerable upper intake level/adverse effects
Calcium	Essential role in blood clotting, muscle con-traction, nerve transmission, and bone and tooth formation	Milk, cheese, yogurt, corn tortillas, calcium-set tofu, Chinese cabbage, kale, broccoli	1,000 mg/day for adults less than 50 years, 1,200 mg/day for adults over 50 years	2,500 mg/day Kidney stones, hypercalce-mia, and renal insufficiency
Chromium	Helps maintain normal blood glu-cose levels	Some cere-als, meats, poultry, fish, beer	No RDA set Adequate intake is 25 μg/day for women, 35 μg/day for men	Not deter-mined Chronic renal failure asso-ciated with excessive con-sumption
Iron	Essential for red blood cell forma-tion	Fruits, veg-etables, meat, poultry, and fortified bread and grain prod-ucts such as cereal	18 mg/day for premenopausal women 8mg/day for men and post-menopausal women	45 mg/day Gastrointestinal disturbances
Magnesium	Participates in enzyme systems, assists in calcium and potassium uptake	Green leafy vegetables, unpolished grains, nuts, meat, starches, milk	320 mg/day for women, 420 mg/day for men	350 mg/day supplements containing magnesium may cause diarrhea

	Function	Food Source	Recommended Dietary Allowance	Tolerable upper intake level/adverse effects
Selenium	Defends against oxidative stress; regulates thyroid hormone actions	Organ meats, seafood, plants	55 µg/day	400 µg/day Hair and nail brittleness and loss
Vanadium	No biological function in humans has been identified	Mushrooms, shellfish, black pepper, parsley, and dill seed	No RDA or adequate intake established	1.8 mg/day Renal lesions
Zinc	Protein synthesis, taste sensitivity, and cell growth	Fortified cereals, red meats, seafood	8 mg/day for women 11 mg/day for men	40 mg/day Interference with the absorption of copper

Water

Most people don't include water in conversations about nutrients, and most people fail to meet their daily water requirements. About 60% of the human body is composed of water. It is needed to help digest food, carry waste from the cells, and control body temperature. The carbohydrates and proteins that our bodies use as food are metabolized and transported by water in the bloodstream. You must replace 2 1/2 quarts of water every day, some through drinking water and the rest taken by the body from the foods you consume.

Chapter 8

Get Movin'

Physical activity is as important to diabetes management as your meal plan and diabetes medications are. Physical activity simply means movement of the body that uses energy. Walking, gardening, briskly pushing a baby stroller while listening to your favorite tune, climbing the stairs, or boogying the night away are all good examples of being active. For health benefits, physical activity should be moderate or vigorous and add up to at least 30 minutes a day. If you can't manage 30 minutes nonstop, you can split up those 30 minutes into several parts. For example, you could take three brisk 10-minute walks, one after each meal.

Benefits of Physical Activity

Research has shown that physical activity can...

- Lower your blood glucose during and after exercise
- Lower your A1C (3 month average of blood sugar levels)
- Lower your blood pressure
- Lower your bad cholesterol and raise your good cholesterol
- Lower your triglycerides
- Improve your body's ability to use insulin
- Lower your risk for heart disease and stroke
- Keep your heart and bones strong
- Keep your joints flexible

- Lower your risk of falling

- Help you lose weight and prevent weight regain

- Reduce your body fat and maintain muscle mass

- Give you more energy

- Reduce your stress

I know these benefits are enough to make you want to start exercising right now, but before you begin any new physical activity, make sure you clear it with your doctor first. If your diabetes is not well controlled or if you have long-term complications of diabetes, such as retinopathy (eye disease), nephropathy (kidney disease), or neuropathy (nerve disease), you need to be careful about the type of exercise you choose. Some exercises can actually make your problems worse. For example, activities that increase the pressure in the blood vessels of your eyes, such as lifting heavy weights, can make diabetic retinopathy worse. Activities such as jogging can cause foot blisters if you already have significant neuropathy involving the feet. Furthermore, people with diabetes frequently have "silent" coronary heart disease which may prevent even moderate exercise in some individuals.

Treating Hypoglycemia

If your blood glucose is 70 mg/dL or lower, have one of the following right away:

- 2 or 3 glucose tablets

- 1/2 cup (4 ounces) of any fruit juice

- 1/2 cup (4 ounces) of a regular (not diet) soft drink

- 1 cup (8 ounces) of milk

- 5 or 6 pieces of hard candy

- 1 or 2 teaspoons of sugar or honey

After 15 minutes, check your blood glucose again. If it's still too low, have another serving. Repeat until your blood glucose is 70 or higher. If it will be an hour or more before your next meal, have a snack as well.

Low Blood Glucose

Increasing your physical activity may cause low blood glucose or hypoglycemia if you are taking insulin or certain diabetes pills, including sulfonylureas and meglitinides. If you are not sure what type of diabetes pills you are taking, ask your health-care team; not all diabetes pills cause low blood glucose.

Hypoglycemia can make you feel shaky, weak, confused, irritable, hungry, or tired. Low blood glucose can happen while you exercise, right afterward, or even up to a day later. For this reason, you should monitor your blood glucose levels closely before and after exercise.

Checking your blood glucose before you exercise will help you decide whether you need a snack that can provide some additional glucose, or fuel, to prevent hypoglycemia during exercise. If your blood glucose is below 100 mg/dL you should have a small snack. If you take insulin, ask your health-care team whether you should change your dosage before you exercise. Keeping a record of your blood glucose readings and exercise will help you develop your own individual exercise and snack guidelines. The following chart can serve as a general guideline to get you started.

Physical Activity and Snack Guidelines			
Intensity	Duration (minutes)	Snack (Carbohydrate grams)	Frequency
Mild-to moderate Walking slowly (1–2 mph), Bowling or vacuuming	<30	May not be needed	___
Moderate Walking briskly (3 ½ mph) Hiking or dancing	30 to 60	15 grams 8 animal crackers or 1 medium piece of fruit	Each hour
High Running, jogging, Aerobics or chopping wood	60+	30 to 50 grams 8 animal crackers plus 1 cup milk or 1 turkey sandwich plus 1 cup milk	Each hour

Additional Safety Guidelines

You should not exercise when your blood glucose is above 300 mg/dl because your level can go even higher. This usually happens because there is not enough insulin to help glucose enter the muscle cells. This lack of glucose in the muscle cells causes the body to make more glucose. This makes your glucose level go higher. It's best not to exercise until your blood glucose is lower. Also, exercise is not recommended if your fasting blood glucose is above 250 and you have ketones in your urine.

- Make sure you exercise in cotton socks and comfortable, well-fitting shoes that are designed for the activity you are doing.

- Check your feet before and after exercise for cuts, sores, bumps, or redness. Call your doctor if any foot problems develop.

- Wear diabetes identification.

- Drink plenty of sugar-free fluid before, during, and after exercise.

- Always carry glucose tablets, hard candy, or juice.

- Exercise with a partner if possible and tell your partner that you have diabetes and what they can do to help you if you have a hypoglycemic reaction.

- If you are exercising alone, tell someone where you will be exercising.

Chapter 9

Monitoring Blood Glucose

Research shows that keeping your blood glucose close to normal reduces your chances of having eye, kidney, and nerve problems. To control your diabetes, you need to know your blood glucose numbers and your goals.

There are two different methods to measure your blood glucose: the A1C test and blood glucose monitoring you do yourself.

The A1C test reflects your average blood glucose level over the last 3 months. In other words, it tells what your blood glucose has been 24/7 for the past 90 days. It is the best way to know your overall blood glucose control during this period of time. This test used to be called hemoglobin A1C or HbA1C. The higher the amount of glucose in your blood, the higher your A1C result will be. A high A1C result will increase your chances for serious health problems.

The process of monitoring one's own blood glucose is often referred to as self-monitoring of blood glucose, or SMBG. The blood glucose monitoring you do yourself uses a drop of blood and a meter that measures the level of glucose in your blood at the time you do the test. Some people need to monitor their glucose levels more often than others do. SMBG is usually done before meals, after meals, and/or at bedtime. For example, you may monitor before break-fast and before lunch on even days, but before dinner and before bed on odd days—or before breakfast and two hours after on even days, and before dinner and two hours after on odd days. The results of your tests can help you manage your diabetes day-by-day or even hour-by-hour. How often you use your glucose meter should be based on the recommendation of your health-care provider. SMBG is recommended for all people with diabetes but especially for those who take insulin.

Optimal Glucose Control	
ADA	**ACE**
A1C scores	
< 7.0%	≤ 6.5%
Fasting glucose*	
90–130 mg/dl	< 110 mg/dl
2-hour post meal glucose	
< 180 mg/dl	< 140 mg/dl
*Fasting—blood glucose first thing in the morning, before eating.	

You and your health-care team need to use both the A1C and SMBG tests to get a complete picture of your blood glucose control.

The American College of endocrinology (ACE) and the American Diabetes Association (ADA) are two major organizations that have set guidelines for optimal blood glucose control to prevent diabetes complications. These guidelines can be found in the chart above. Your individual goals should be set with your health-care team.

Diabetes medication, food, and activity all affect your blood glucose levels. Most people think that food is the only factor that needs to be adjusted when trying to achieve glycemic control. Yes, food may be of primary concern if you are overeating. But if you are eating a well-balanced, low-calorie diet, and you are still not meeting your target glucose levels, you should consider talking to your health-care provider. You may need to change the timing or type of your diabetes medication. You may also benefit from an increase in your physical activity, or if you are exercising, a change in when you exercise may help. Additionally, a change in the distribution of your food may help as well. In Chapter 11, "The Choice is Yours," you will learn how to distribute your food based on carbohydrate counting.

Part III

Eating Soulfully and Healthfully: Engaging the Enemy

Chapter 10

The Diabetes Soul Food Pyramid

On April 19, 2005, the United States Department of Agriculture (USDA) released MyPyramid, which replaces the Food Guide Pyramid introduced in 1992. The new MyPyramid is part of an overall food guidance system that emphasizes the need for a more individualized approach to improving diet and lifestyle. MyPyramid represents the recommended proportion of foods from each food group, and focuses on the importance of making smart food choices in every food group, every day.

Like MyPyramid, the Diabetes Soul Food Pyramid was developed to offer African Americans and consumers of traditional foods from the South and the Caribbean, an individualized approach to improving diet and lifestyle. The key message of the Diabetes Soul Food Pyramid is that you don't have to give up ethnic food but simply learn how to place it in your diet successfully.

The Diabetes Soul Food Pyramid maintains the shape of the original Food Guide Pyramid but groups foods together based on their carbohydrate content, rather than their classification as a food. For example, you will find black-eyed peas and sweet potatoes in the grain group instead of the vegetable group. Cheese will be found in the meat group instead of the milk group. A serving of vegetable is 1 1/2 cup in the Diabetes Soul Food Pyramid and 1/2 cup in MyPyramid. A serving of rice or pasta is 1/3 cup in the Diabetes Soul Food Pyramid and 1/2 cup in MyPyramid. Fruit juice is 1/2 cup in the Diabetes Soul Food Pyramid and 3/4 cup in MyPyramid. In the Diabetes Soul Food Pyramid, all foods containing carbohydrates are proportioned so that they will provide about 15 grams of carbohydrates.

In Chapter 11, you will learn how to use the Diabetes Soul Food Pyramid to manage your diabetes successfully.

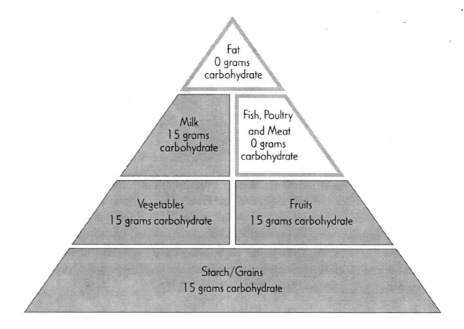

Chapter 11

The Choice Is Yours

In a perfect world, everyone who has been diagnosed with diabetes would have the opportunity to meet at least once with a registered dietitian for an individualized meal plan. But if you are like the vast majority of people with diabetes, you probably received very vague instruction that only served as a source of frustration and stress. Statements like "Just stay away from sugar," "Lose some weight," "Don't eat fat," or "Eat smaller portions" are all too common. And worse yet, you might have been given one of those famous tear-off sheets with no explanation or regard for your cultural or ethnic food preferences.

Well, let me take this opportunity to congratulate you. *Say what?* Yes, I want to congratulate you. Even if you skipped all the other chapters and turned to this one first, it is clear you realized there's more to managing diabetes than simply "avoiding sugar." How right you are! Meal planning and changing eating behavior is one of the most difficult areas of diabetes self-management. Consideration must be given to every aspect of your lifestyle, your willingness, and your ability to make changes. And now that I've validated your feelings of past frustration, let's start with some basic facts.

As you discovered in Chapter 7, everything that you eat, with the exception of pure animal protein and fat, has some carbohydrate content. When you eat foods containing carbohydrates, like corn bread, grits, peaches, milk, or even collard greens, your body breaks these foods down into sugar called glucose. The glucose then enters into your bloodstream, where it can be utilized to energize the cells of the body. The more carbohydrate-containing foods you eat at a meal, the more glucose will enter the bloodstream.

Now remember, in type 2 diabetes, your body does not produce enough insulin to take the glucose out of the bloodstream and allow it to be used for energy, or you have enough insulin, but the insulin is unable to do its job properly (insulin resistance). It's often said that a picture is worth a thousand words, so to better understand what's going on in your body and why you need to change the way you eat, picture this...

We have all experienced a clogged drain at one time or another. If you have a clogged drain and water is slowly dripping down the drain, it is not obvious that the drain is clogged. If you turn the faucet on high and fill the sink up with water, though, it takes a very long time for that water level to go down. *Or in the worst-case scenario, it won't move at all.* This is basically what happens in your body as a result of insulin resistance. If you eat small amounts of foods containing carbohydrates at a meal (like the drips of water in the clogged drain), your body will work more efficiently. Your blood glucose levels will not go up as high.

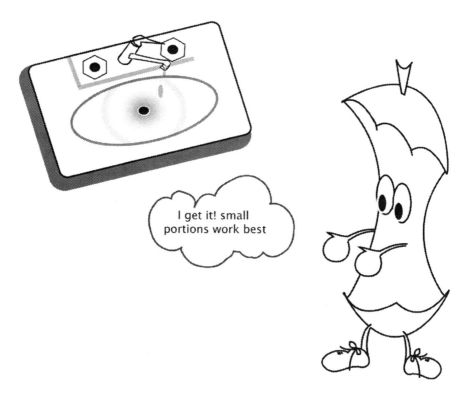

On the other hand, if you chow down on some corn bread, potato salad, maca-roni and cheese, and sweet potatoes all in one meal…well that's like turning the faucet on high. Your glucose levels are going to go up very high and take a long time to return to normal. To make matters worse, before there is a sig-nificant drop in your glucose levels, you get hungry and eat again. The result? Your glucose levels will rise even higher.

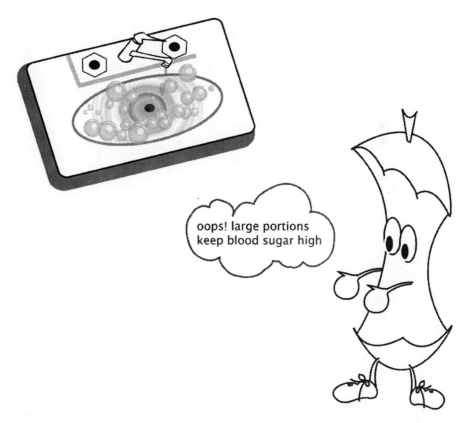

oops! large portions
keep blood sugar high

Now don't misunderstand: this does not mean you can never ever indulge in a piece of warm, made-from-scratch, mouth-watering corn bread. But you cer-tainly must monitor your portions and consider the carbohydrate content. This brings us to meal planning using carbohydrate-counting and the Diabetes Soul Food Pyramid. Experts tell us that it is the total amount of carbohydrates eaten at a meal, and not the source or type, that impacts glucose control. So whether you choose to count each gram of carbohydrate in your food or use the "choice method" of carbohydrate counting, you will learn to include a variety of your favorite foods and maintain good glucose control.

The Choice Method of Carbohydrate Counting

The Diabetes Soul Food Pyramid is a great place to start when using the choice method for counting carbohydrates. Take a look at the Diabetes Soul Food Pyramid on page 48. A carbohydrate choice is a serving of food from the starch, fruit, vegetable, or milk group. Foods in the pyramid that have carbohydrates are found in the shaded boxes. Each serving counts as one carbohydrate choice and gives you 15 grams of carbohydrates. Listed below are some examples of soul food choices found in each food group. Chapters 13–20 provide you with a more extensive listing of foods from each category of the pyramid. And if you like Caribbean, Cajun, or Creole cuisine, you will find your favorites are included. You will also find a two-week soul food menu plan in Appendix A.

Starch

1/2 c grits

1 biscuit (2 1/2" across)

cornbread (2" square)

1/2 c lima beans, black-eyed peas, or succotash

1/3 c yam, sweet potato, or rice

Vegetables

1 1/2 c cooked kale, poke salad, collard greens, or turnips

Fruit

1 medium peach, apple, or orange

1 1/4 c watermelon

17 muscadines or 15 grapes

1/2 c orange or grapefruit juice

Milk

1 c milk

1 c buttermilk

1/2 c evaporated milk

3/4 c fortified soy milk

It is reasonable for most adults to consume 3–4 carbohydrate choices at each meal and eat 1–2 carbohydrate choices for snacks. Look at the table below to determine your best choices. To further determine your best choices, check your blood glucose levels 2 hours after eating a meal. A blood glucose level less than 140 mg/dl, 2 hours after a meal, is an indicator of good diabetes control. If you are not achieving your goals, see a registered dietitian or certified diabetes educator, who will help you find your best choices.

Carbohydrate Choices Per Meal			
	To Lose Weight	To Control Weight	For Active Individuals
Women	3–4	4–5	5–6
Men	4–5	5–6	6–7

If snacks are desired, subtract carbohydrate choices from a meal.

Source: American Diabetes Association.

To determine what a serving size is, you will need to measure your food. I know that sounds like a lot of work, but as in every aspect of life, *you get what you pay for,* and the payoff will be good blood glucose control. If you are still unhappy about the idea of measuring your food, then at least aim for what I call "repeatability." In other words, always use the same cups, dishes, utensils, etc., for the same foods. If you fill your favorite Tupperware bowl with cereal every morning, and your blood glucose levels 2 hours after breakfast are continually higher than your target, try filling that same favorite Tupperware bowl half full. Just remember, the most accurate method of controlling portions is to use measuring cups and spoons. When you measure your food at home, it also makes it easier to choose correct portions when away from home. In "Size Does Matter," Chapter 13, you will learn more about weighing, measuring, and estimating portions.

There will be times when you are eating packaged foods that contain more or less than 15 grams of carbohydrates. The chart below will show you how to convert these foods into carbohydrate choices. Remember, 15 grams of carbohydrate equals 1 carbohydrate choice.

Converting Carbohydrate Grams to Carbohydrate Choices	
Carbohydrate Grams	**Carbohydrate Choices**
0–5	0
6–10	1/2
11–20	1
21–25	1 1/2
26–35	2
36–40	2 1/2
41–50	3
51–55	3 1/2
56–65	4
66–70	4 1/2
71–80	5
Source: American Diabetes Association	

The Gram Method of Carbohydrate Counting

Counting carbohydrates by grams is a more precise method of controlling your carbohydrate intake than the choice method. I find this method gives you greater flexibility, especially when eating prepackaged foods. See the table below to determine your suggested carbohydrate gram intake.

<u>Carbohydrate Grams Per Meal</u>			
	To Lose Weight	To Control Weight	For Active Individuals
Women	45–60	60–75	75–90
Men	60–75	75–90	90–105
If snacks are desired, subtract carbohydrate grams from a meal.			
Source: American Diabetes Association			

To truly master carbohydrate counting, you will need to learn how to read the nutrition facts panel found on food labels.

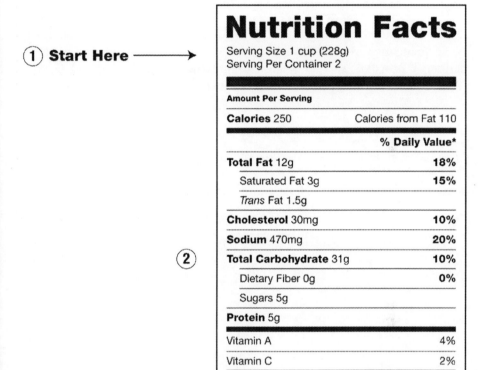

Sample label for
Macaroni & Cheese

The nutrition facts information show you what a serving size is and how many grams of carbohydrates that serving will give you. The nutrition facts panel has a great deal of information on it. For now, we will examine only the information that will assist with carbohydrate counting.

Look at the sample label for macaroni and cheese. (For the purpose of illustration, this is a simplified label.) Starting at the top, look at the serving size; it is 1 cup. There are 2 servings per container. Next, the "Amount Per Serving" will tell you the amount of calories and nutrients in a single serving. At number 2, you will notice that the total carbohydrates (found in bold print) is 31 grams.

One cup of macaroni and cheese has 31 grams of carbohydrates. In lighter print directly under "Total Carbohydrate," you will notice Dietary Fiber and Sugar. The fiber and sugar grams are included in the total grams of carbohydrate. If a food item contains sugar alcohol, it will be listed here also. Remember, it is the total amount of carbohydrates that impacts your glucose levels. Now, for those of you who have been told "Just stay away from sugar"—think about that advice. The sugar content in the macaroni and cheese is 5 grams, counted as part of the total carbohydrates. If your focus is only on the sugar, there will be 26 grams of carbohydrates you didn't count. Moreover, the 26 grams of carbohydrate will make your glucose level rise higher than anticipated. Get the idea? Controlling total carbohydrates is the key to success.

Chapter 12

Label Lingo

Are nutrition labels really helpful? You bet! The nutrition label can help you make quick, informed food choices that contribute to a healthy diet. Although people know they should read the nutrition label, many don't. Typically, it's because they find the information too confusing. The following guidance will demystify the label and help you use the information on the label more effectively and easily.

Sample label for
Macaroni & Cheese

① **Start Here** ⟶

②

③ **Limit these
Nutrients**

④ **Get Enough
of these
Nutrients**

⑤ **Footnote**

Nutrition Facts

Serving Size 1 cup (228g)
Serving Per Container 2

Amount Per Serving

Calories 250   Calories from Fat 110

% Daily Value*

Total Fat 12g	**18%**
Saturated Fat 3g	**15%**
Trans Fat 1.5g	
Cholesterol 30mg	**10%**
Sodium 470mg	**20%**
Total Carbohydrate 31g	**10%**
Dietary Fiber 0g	**0%**
Sugars 5g	
Protein 5g	
Vitamin A	4%
Vitamin C	2%
Calcium	20%
Iron	4%

* Percent Daily Values are based on a 2,000 calorie diet. Your Daily Values may be higher or lower depending on your calorie needs:

	Calories:	2,000	2,500
Total Fat	Less than	65g	80g
Sat Fat	Less than	20g	25g
Cholesterol	Less than	300mg	300mg
Sodium	Less than	2,400mg	2,400mg
Total Carbohydrate		300g	375g
Dietary Fiber		25g	30g

1. The first place to start when you look at the nutrition label is the serving size and number of servings in the package. Serving sizes are based on the amount typically eaten. However, that is not to say that what you consider a serving is the same as a typical serving. Pay attention to the serving size, including how many servings there are in the food package, and compare it to how much you actually eat. In the sample label, a serving is one cup. If you ate the whole package, you would eat two cups. That doubles the calories and other nutrient numbers.

2. The calorie information tells you the number of calories in a single serving and how many calories come from fat. In our sample label, there are 250 calories per serving and 110 calories from fat. That means that about half of the calories come from fat.

3. Fat, cholesterol, and sodium should be limited in the diet. Too much of these nutrients can increase your risk of certain chronic diseases, like heart disease, some cancers, or high blood pressure. To keep your intake as low as possible, make sure the "% Daily Value" of these nutrients is less than 5%. (Another easy way to keep your fat intake low is to aim for no more than 3 grams of total fat per 100 calories.)

4. You should try to get enough essential nutrients like calcium, iron, and vitamins A and C, as well as other components such as dietary fiber. Try to average 100% for each one of these nutrients each day. A food item with 20% or more of these essential nutrients is high in those nutrients. In the sample, the daily value for calcium is 20%, which means the macaroni and cheese is high in calcium.

5. The footnote is only found on larger packages and provides general dietary information about important nutrients. When the full footnote does appear, it will always be the same. It doesn't change from product to product because it shows dietary advice for all Americans; it is not about a specific food product.

As you can see, the nutrition label is very helpful. It can help you make informed decisions and manage your dietary intake for optimal health.

Nutrient Content Claims

The Nutrition Labeling and Education Act of 1990 permits the use of label claims that characterize the level of a nutrient in a food. Nutrient claims describe the level of a nutrient or dietary substance in the product, using terms such as "free," "high," and "low." Or they compare the level of a nutrient in a food to that of another food, using terms such as "more," "reduced," and "lite." Sound confusing? Here are some tips that will help you make sense of it all.

Nutrition Content Claims

Free	
Fat-free	less than 0.5 grams (g) of fat per serving
Cholesterol-free	less than 2 milligrams (mg) of cholesterol per serving
Sodium-free	less than 5 milligrams (mg) of sodium per serving
Sugar-free	less than 0.5 grams (g) of sugar per serving
Calorie-free	less than 5 calories per serving
Low	
Low fat	3 grams (g) of fat or less per serving
Low saturated fat	1 gram of saturated fat or less per serving
Low cholesterol	20 milligrams (mg) of cholesterol or less per serving
Low sodium	140 milligrams (mg) of sodium or less per serving
Low calorie	40 calories or less per serving
Reduced or **Less**	
Reduced or Less fat	at least 25% less fat than the regular food
Reduced or Less saturated fat	at least 25% less saturated fat than the regular food
Reduced or Less cholesterol	at least 25% less cholesterol than the regular food
Reduced or Less sodium	at least 25% less sodium than the regular food

Reduced or Less sugar	at least 25% less sugar than the regular food
Reduced or Less calories	at least 25% fewer calories than the regular food
Light or **Lite**	1/3 fewer calories or 50% less fat than the regular food

Chapter 13

Size Does Matter

How much are you really eating, one portion or one serving? Most people are confused when it comes to portions and servings, often using the terms interchangeably. The fact is, portions and servings are two completely different measurements.

A portion is the amount of food you *choose* to eat for dinner, snack, or any eating occasion. Portions, of course, can be bigger or smaller than the recommended food servings. A serving is a unit of measure used to describe the amount of food *recommended* from each food group. It is the amount of food listed on the Nutrition Facts panel on packaged food or the amount of food recommended in MyPyramid and the Dietary Guidelines for Americans. For example, if you're counting carbohydrate choices or grams, and you don't know what a serving is, you will get more or even less carbohydrates than you're aiming for. This mistake could result in an elevation in your blood sugar, or your blood sugar may go too low. Successful management of your diabetes requires a good understanding of serving sizes and how to properly weigh and measure your foods, particularly foods containing carbohydrates.

People often think that because they've dieted in the past, they know what a serving is. The truth is, the longer it's been since you actually used a measuring cup, measuring spoons, and scale, the greater the chance your portion is going to be too large.

Using measuring utensils at home can bring you back to reality and help you judge the correct portion size for your meals when eating out. But for those of you who find it impossible, for one reason or another, to weigh and measure anything, the chart below provides a number of ways you can at least "guesstimate" your servings.

Another way to determine how much you're eating is the "repeatability" method. With this method, you only need to measure your food one time. For example, measure a serving size of your favorite cereal and pour it into a bowl. The next time you eat cereal, use the same bowl and fill it to the same level.

Serving Size Guide

One Portion of...	One Serving Looks Like a...
Grain/Starch Products	
1 cup of cereal flakes	closed fist
1 pancake	compact disc
1/2 cup of cooked rice, pasta, or potato	1/2 baseball
1 slice of bread	cassette tape
1 piece of corn bread	bar of soap
1/2 cup beans	1/2 baseball
4 small cookies	4 casino chips
Vegetables and Fruits	
1 cup of salad greens	baseball
1/2 cup cooked vegetables	1/2 baseball
1 baked potato	closed fist
1 med fruit	baseball
1/4 cup of raisins	large egg
Dairy and Cheese	
1 1/2 oz. cheese	4 stacked dice or a C battery
1/2 cup of ice cream	1/2 baseball
Meat and Alternatives	
3 oz. meat, fish, and poultry	deck of cards
3 oz. grilled/baked fish	checkbook
2 Tbsp. peanut butter	ping-pong ball or roll of film
Fats	
1 tsp. margarine or spreads	tip of thumb

Chapter 14

Upscale Soul Food Dining

Soul food has gone mainstream, no longer confined to the good old finger-lickin', down-home, mom-and-pop eateries of the South. Fine soul food dining can be experienced in every major city. The tips below can help make your upscale soul food dining experience a healthy one.

Menu Item	Healthy Choice	Avoid or order with caution
Appetizers	Steamed, boiled, or marinated seafood Tomato or vegetable juice (limit, high in salt) Broth, bouillon, or consommé (limit, high in salt), black-eyed pea soup	High-Fat items such as fried and breaded buffalo sticks, buffalo wings, blue cheese dip, fritters, fried catfish, fried green tomatoes or fried plantain Cream soups (high in fat and salt)
Salads	Tossed greens (Ask for dressing on the side) Vinaigrette or low-calorie dressing	Croutons, potato, and pasta salads (high in fat and carbohydrates) Coleslaw, chicken, or seafood salads (high in fat) Creamy or cheese type dressing, Caesar salad

Menu Item	Healthy Choice	Avoid or order with caution
	Low-calorie extras, like mushrooms, peppers, onions	High-calorie, high-carbohydrate extras, like bacon bits, fried meats, guacamole, cheese, or croutons
Entrees	Baked, broiled, black-ened, Cajun, or mari-nated (limit, high in salt), jerk, grilled, poached, steamed, stir-fried, cooked in its own juice	Breaded, fried, in or with cheese sauce, cream sauce, or gravy. Parmesan, au gratin, escalloped, battered fried, or corn-flour crusted
	Ask for sauce on the side Remove skin and visible fat	Sweet and sour, honey-glazed, honey mustard, BBQ, (high in carbohydrates)
Side Orders	Steamed, grilled, or roasted vegetables, rice, boiled potatoes, small baked sweet potato	Sweet potato fries, mashed potato with gravy and/or butter, maca-roni and cheese
Desserts	Fresh fruit, 1/2 cup low-fat frozen yogurt or ice cream, angel food cake	Sweet potato pie, ice cream with topping, cheese cake, carrot cake, red velvet cake, or cobbler

Dining Out Game Plan

♦ Choose a restaurant that offers a varied menu with healthy alternatives.

♦ Avoid buffets and "all you can eat" restaurants.

♦ Know what you want to order before you go to the restaurant—this can help overcome impulse ordering.

♦ Have a generic plan (if all else fails, order "fish of the day").

♦ Make shrimp cocktail your main course and fill in with à la carte vegetables.

♦ Know your meal plan and think before you order.

♦   Ask how the food is prepared.

♦   Don't be afraid to make special requests.

♦   Check your blood sugar two hours after your meal.

Part IV

More Soul Food Choices:
Staying on Track

Chapter 15

Starch Choices

The starch group includes bagels, bread, muffins, cereals, crackers, grains, noodles, starchy vegetables, roots, and tubers. For a healthy diet, eat at least 3 oz of whole-grain products per day. Make at least half of the total grains eaten whole grains, such as brown rice, buckwheat, bulgur, oatmeal, wild rice, whole-wheat bread, crackers, pasta, and tortillas. One ounce is about 1 slice of bread, about 1 cup of breakfast cereal, or 1/2 cup of cooked rice, cereal, or pasta.

The Dietary Guidelines suggest you eat a total of 6 oz of starches every day.

Starch Tips:

- Eat fewer fried and high-fat starches, such as regular biscuits, corn bread, dressing, pancakes, stuffing, or waffles.

- Limit additional butter, margarines, mayonnaise, shortening, and oil

- Check the ingredient list on grain product labels. For whole-grain products, you will see the words "whole" or "whole-grain" before the grain ingredient's name.

- Check the Nutrition Facts label for the fiber content of food products. Fiber content is a good clue to the amount of whole grain in the product.

STARCH CHOICES

	Portion	Cal	Fat (g)	Sat Fat (g)	Carb (g)	Fiber (g)	Sod (mgs)	Carb Choices	Exchanges
Bagels									
Plain 4"	1	245	1	0.2	48	2	475	3	3 Starch
Cinnamon-raisin 4"	1	244	2	0.2	49	2	287	3	3 Starch
Biscuits									
Homemade with 2% milk, 2 1/2"	1	212	10	2.6	27	0.9	348	2	1 Starch, 2 Fat
Refrigerated dough, regular 2 1/2"	1	93	4	1	13	0.4	325	1	1 Starch, 1 Fat
Refrigerated dough, low-fat 2 1/4"	1	63	0.3	0.6	12	0.4	305	1	1 Starch
Breads									
Bammy	1	217	Tr	0	53.5	0	325	3 1/2	3 1/2 Starch
Corn bread, 3 3/4"×2 1/2" ×3/4"	1	188	6	1.6	29	1.4	467	2	2 Starch, 1 Fat
Cracked wheat bread	1 slice	65	1	0.2	12	1.4	135	1	1 Starch
Egg bread, challah	1/2" slice	115	2	0.6	19	0.9	197	1	1 Starch
French or Vienna (includes sourdough)	1/2" slice	69	1	0.2	13	0.8	152	1	1 Starch
Hard dough bread	1 thin slice	261	2.3	-	50.2	0.2	431	3	3 Starch
Italian	1 slice	54	1	0.2	10	0.5	117	1	1 Starch

	Portion	Cal	Fat (g)	Sat Fat (g)	Carb (g)	Fiber (g)	Sod (mgs)	Carb Choices	Exchanges
Mixed grain	1 slice	65	1	0.2	12	1.7	127	1	1 Starch
Oatmeal	1 slice	73	1	0.2	13	1.1	162	1	1 Starch
Pita, 4"	1	77	Tr	Tr	16	0.6	150	1	1 Starch
Pita, 6-1/2"	1	165	1	0.1	33	1.3	322	2	1 Starch
Pumpernickel	1 slice	80	1	0.1	15	2.1	225	1	1 Starch
Raisin	1 slice	71	1	0.3	14	1.1	101	1	1 Starch
Rye	1 slice	83	1	0.2	15	1.9	211	1	1 Starch
Tortilla, corn, 6" diameter	1	58	1	0.1	12	1.4	42	1	1 Starch
Tortilla, flour, 6" diameter	1	104	2	0.6	18	1.1	153	1	1 Starch
Wheat	1 slice	65	1	0.2	12	1.1	133	1	1 Starch
Wheat, reduced-calorie	1 slice	46	1	0.1	10	2.8	118	1/2	1/2 Starch
White	1 slice	67	1	0.1	12	0.6	135	1	1 Starch
White, reduced-calorie	1 slice	48	1	0.1	10	2.2	104	1/2	1/2 Starch
Whole wheat	1 slice	69	1	0.3	13	1.9	148	1	1 Starch
Misc. Bread Products									
Bread crumbs									
Dry, grated, plain, enriched	1 oz	112	2	0.3	21	0.7	244	1 1/2	1 1/2 Starch
Soft crumbs	1 cup	120	2	0.2	22	1	242	1 1/2	1 1/2 Starch
Bread dressing/ stuffing									
Corn bread, homemade	1/2 cup	179	8.8	1.8	21.9	2.9	455	1 1/2	1 1/2 Starch, 2 Fat

	Portion	Cal	Fat (g)	Sat Fat (g)	Carb (g)	Fiber (g)	Sod (mgs)	Carb Choices	Exchanges
Prepared from dry mix	1/2 cup	178	9	1.7	22	2.9	543	1 1/2	1 1/2 Starch, 2 Fat
Bread sticks 4" × 1/2"	1 stick	21	0	0	3	0	33	0	1/4 Starch
Croissant, butter	1 medium	231	12	6.6	26	1.5	424	2	2 Starch, 2 Fat
Croutons, seasoned	1 cup	186	7	2.1	25	2	495	1 1/2	1 1/2 Starch
English muffin	1	134	1	0.1	26	1.5	264	2	2 Starch
French toast	1 slice	151	7.4	2	16.2	0	310	1	1 Starch, 1 1/2 Fat
Hamburger bun	1	123	2	0.5	22	1.2	241	1 1/2	1 1/2 Starch
Hotdog bun	1	123	2	0.5	22	1.2	241	1 1/2	1 1/2 Starch
Muffins									
Blueberry, prepared from mix	1 small	150	4	0.7	24	0.6	219	1 1/2	1 1/2 Starch
Bran	1 small	138	5	1.2	23	2.1	234	1 1/2	1 1/2 Starch, 1 Fat
Corn, prepared from mix	1 small	161	5	1.4	25	1.2	398	1 1/2	1 ½ Starch, 1 Fat
Naan 8" × 2"	1/4	80	1	0	15	ND	ND	1	1 Starch
Rolls									
Brown and serve	1	84	2	0.5	14	1	146	1	1 Starch
Dinner	1	84	2	0.5	14	0.8	146	1	1 Starch
Hard, kaiser	1	167	2	0.3	30	1.3	310	2	2 Starch

	Portion	Cal	Fat (g)	Sat Fat (g)	Carb (g)	Fiber (g)	Sod (mgs)	Carb Choices	Exchanges
Tea type breads									
Banana bread	2 oz slice	196	6	1.3	33	0.7	181	2	2 Starch, 1 Fat
Pumpkin bread	2 oz slice	223	2.5	0	45	1.3	327	3	3 Starch
Cereal Bars									
Breakfast Bar, cereal crust w/fruit filling, fat-free	1	121	Tr	Tr	28	0.8	203	2	2 Starch
Nutri-Grain cereal bar, fruit-filled	1 bar	136	3	0.6	27	0.8	110	2	1 1/2 Starch, 1/2 Fat
Hot Cereals									
Cooked Corn (Hominy) Grits									
White	1 cup	145	Tr	0.1	31	0.5	0	2	2 Starch
Yellow	1 cup	145	Tr	0.1	31	0.5	0	2	2 Starch
Instant, plain	1 packet	89	Tr	Tr	21	1.2	289	1 1/2	1 1/2 Starch
Cream of Wheat									
Regular	1 cup	133	1	0.1	29	1.8	3	2	2 Starch
Quick	1 cup	129	Tr	0.1	27	1.2	139	2	2 Starch
Oat Bran	1 cup	87	2	0.4	25	5.7	2.2	1 1/2	1 Starch
Oatmeal, instant, fortified, plain	1 packet	104	2	0.3	18	3	285	1	1 Starch

	Portion	Cal	Fat (g)	Sat Fat (g)	Carb (g)	Fiber (g)	Sod (mgs)	Carb Choices	Exchanges
Quaker Oats, instant									
Apples and Cinnamon	1 packet	125	1	0.3	26	2.5	121	2	2 Starch
Maple and Brown Sugar	1 packet	153	2	0.4	31	2.6	234	2	2 Starch
Wheatena	1 cup	136	1	0.2	29	6.6	5	2	2 Starch
Ready-To-Eat Cereals									
All-Bran	1/2 cup	79	1	0.2	23	9.7	61	1 1/2	1 1/2 Starch
Apple Jacks	1 cup	116	Tr	0.1	27	0.6	134	2	2 Starch
Basic 4	1 cup	201	3	0.4	42	3.4	323	3	3 Starch, 1/2 Fat
Bran Flakes, Kellogg's	1 cup	127	0.9	0	31	6.2	304	2	1 1/2 Starch
Ready-To-Eat Cereals									
Cap'n Crunch	3/4 cup	107	1	0.4	23	0.9	208	1 1/2	1 1/2 Starch
Cap'n Crunch's Crunchberries	3/4 cup	104	1	0.3	22	0.6	190	1 1/2	1 1/2 Starch
Cap'n Crunch's Peanut Butter Crunch	3/4 cup	112	2	0.5	22	0.8	204	1 1/2	1 1/2 Starch
Cheerios	1 cup	110	2	0.4	23	2.6	284	1 1/2	1 1/2 Starch
Cheerios, Apple Cinnamon	3/4 cup	118	2	0.3	25	1.6	150	1 1/2	1 1/2 Starch

	Portion	Cal	Fat (g)	Sat Fat (g)	Carb (g)	Fiber (g)	Sod (mgs)	Carb Choices	Exchanges
Cheerios, Honey Nut	1 cup	115	1	0.2	24	1.6	259	1 1/2	1 1/2 Starch
Chex, Corn	1 cup	113	Tr	0.1	26	0.5	289	2	2 Starch
Chex, Honey Nut	3/4 cup	117	1	0.1	26	0.4	224	2	2 Starch
Chex, Multi-Bran	1 cup	165	1	0.2	41	6.4	325	3	3 Starch
Chex, Rice	1 1/4 cup	117	Tr	Tr	27	0.3	291	2	2 Starch
Chex, Wheat	1 cup	104	1	0.1	24	3.3	269	1 1/2	1 1/2 Starch
Cinnamon Toast Crunch	3/4 cup	124	3	0.5	24	1.5	210	1 1/2	1 1/2 Starch, 1/2 Fat
Cocoa Krispies	3/4 cup	120	1	0.6	27	0.4	210	2	2 Starch
Cocoa Puffs	1 cup	119	1	0.2	27	0.2	181	2	2 Starch
Complete Wheat Bran Flakes	3/4 cup	95	1	0.1	23	4.6	226	1 1/2	1 1/2 Starch
Corn Flakes, Kellogg's	1 cup	102	Tr	0.1	24	0.8	298	1 1/2	1 1/2 Starch
Corn Flakes, Total	1 1/3 cup	112	Tr	0.2	26	0.8	203	1 1/2	1 1/2 Starch
Corn Pops	1 cup	118	Tr	0.1	28	0.4	123	2	2 Starch
Crispix	1 cup	108	Tr	0.1	25	0.6	240	1 1/2	1 1/2 Starch
Froot Loops	1 cup	117	1	0.4	26	0.6	141	2	2 Starch
Frosted Flakes	3/4 cup	119	Tr	0.1	28	0.6	200	2	2 Starch
Frosted Mini-Wheats									
Regular	1 cup	173	1	0.2	42	5.5	2	3	3 Starch
Bite Size	1 cup	187	1	0.2	45	5.9	2	3	3 Starch

	Portion	Cal	Fat (g)	Sat Fat (g)	Carb (g)	Fiber (g)	Sod (mgs)	Carb Choices	Exchanges
Golden Grahams	3/4 cup	116	1	0.2	26	0.9	275	2	2 Starch
Ready-To-Eat Cereals									
Honey Nut Clusters	1 cup	213	3	0.4	43	4.2	239	3	3 Starch, 1/2 Fat
Kashi Good Friends	1 cup	170	2	0	43	12	130	3	3 Starch
Kix	1 1/3 cup	114	1	0.2	26	0.8	263	2	2 Starch
Kix, Berry Berry	3/4 cup	120	1	0.2	26	0.2	185	2	2 Starch
Life	3/4 cup	121	1	0.2	25	2	174	1 1/2	1 1/2 Starch
Life, Cinnamon	1 cup	190	2	0.3	40	3	220	2 1/2	2 1/2 Starch
Lucky Charms	1 cup	116	1	0.2	25	1.2	203	1 1/2	1 1/2 Starch
Nature Valley Granola	3/4 cup	248	10	1.3	36	3.5	89	2 1/2	2 1/2 Starch, 2 Fat
Granola with raisins, low-fat	1/2 cup	195	3	0.8	40	3	129	2 1/2	2 1/2 Starch, 1/2 Fat
Product 19	1 cup	110	Tr	Tr	25	1	216	1 1/2	1 1/2 Starch
Puffed Rice	1 cup	56	Tr	Tr	13	0.2	Tr	1	1 Starch
Puffed Wheat	1 cup	44	Tr	Tr	10	0.5	Tr	1/2	1/2 Starch
Raisin Bran	1 cup	178	1	0.2	43	5	240	3	3 Starch
Raisin Nut Bran	1 cup	209	4	0.7	41	5.1	246	3	3 Starch
Rice Krispies	1 1/4 cup	124	Tr	0.1	29	0.4	354	2	2 Starch
Shredded Wheat	2 biscuits	156	1	0.1	38	5.3	3	2 1/2	2 1/2 Starch
Special K	1 cup	115	Tr	0	22	1	250	1 1/2	1 1/2 Starch

	Portion	Cal	Fat (g)	Sat Fat (g)	Carb (g)	Fiber (g)	Sod (mgs)	Carb Choices	Exchanges
Total, Whole-Grain	3/4 cup	105	1	0.2	24	2.6	199	1 1/2	1 1/2 Starch
Trix	1 cup	122	2	0.4	26	0.7	197	2	2 Starch
Wheaties	1 cup	110	1	0.2	24	2.1	222	1 1/2	1 1/2 Starch
Wheaties, Honey-Frosted	3/4 cup	110	Tr	0.1	26	1.5	211	2	2 Starch
Crackers									
Animal crackers	23 pcs(2oz)	254	7.9	2	42.2	0.6	224	3	3 Starch, 1 1/2 Fat
Cheese Nips	20 pieces	140	6	1.5	19	0	340	1	1 Starch, 1 Fat
Goldfish, all varieties	50 pieces	127	5.5	1.8	17	0.5	209	1	1 Starch, 1 Fat
Graham, crushed	1 cup	355	8	1.3	65	2.4	508	4	4 Starch, 1 1/2 Fat
Graham, plain 2 1/2" square	2 squares	59	1	0.2	11	0.4	85	1	1 Starch
Harvest Crisp	13 crackers	140	4.5	1.0	22	1	300	1 1/2	1 1/2 Starch
Matzo, plain	1 matzo	112	Tr	0.1	24	0.9	1	1 1/2	1 1/2 Starch
Melba rounds	4 crackers	78	0.6	0	15.3	1.3	4	1	1 Starch
Melba toast, plain	4 pieces	78	1	0.1	15	1.3	166	1	1 Starch
Oyster type	1 cup	195	5	1.3	32	1.4	586	2	2 Starch, 1 Fat
Peanut-butter filled crackers	2 crackers	34	1.7	0.4	4.1	0.2	66	0	1/3 Starch
Ritz	1 cracker	79	3.7	0.6	10.3	0.3	124	1/2	1/2 Starch

	Portion	Cal	Fat (g)	Sat Fat (g)	Carb (g)	Fiber (g)	Sod (mgs)	Carb Choices	Exchanges
Rye wafer, whole-grain, plain	1 wafer	37	Tr	Tr	9	2.5	87	1/2	1/2 Starch
Saltine, square	4 crackers	52	1	0.4	9	0.4	156	1/2	1/2 Starch
Saltine, unsalted top	4 crackers	52	1.4	0.4	8.6	0.4	76	1/2	1/2 Starch
Sandwich, wheat with cheese	1	33	1	0.4	4	0.1	98	0	1/3 Starch
Triscuit	5 crackers	107	4.3	0.7	15	2.1	114	1	1 Starch, 1/2 Fat
Wheat Thins	16 crackers	136	5.8	0.9	20	0.9	168	1	1 Starch
Zwieback	1 toast	35	1	0	6	0	10	1/2	1/3 Starch
Grains									
Arrowroot flour	3 Tbsp	80	0	0	20	0	0	1	1 Starch
Banana flour, commercial	3 Tbsp	81	0.4	0.2	21	0.4	1	1 1/2	1 1/2 Starch
Barley, dry	1 cup	704	2	0.5	155	31.2	18	10 1/2	10 Starch
Barley, cooked	1 cup	193	1	0.1	44	6	5	3	3 Starch
Bulgur, dry	1 cup	479	2	0.3	106	25.6	24	7	7 Starch
Bulgur, cooked	1 cup	151	Tr	0.1	34	8.2	9	2	2 Starch
Carob flour	1 cup	229	1	0.1	92	41	36	6	6 Starch
Cassava, fresh root, cooked	1/2 cup	110	0.2	0	27	1.3	9	2	2 Starch
Cornmeal, dry, whole grain	1 cup	442	4	0.6	94	8.9	43	6 1/2	6 1/2 Starch

	Portion	Cal	Fat (g)	Sat Fat (g)	Carb (g)	Fiber (g)	Sod (mgs)	Carb Choices	Exchanges
Cornmeal, degermed, enriched	1 cup	505	2	0.3	107	10.2	4	7	6 Starch
Cornstarch	1 Tbsp	30	Tr	Tr	7	0.1	1	.1/2	7 Starch
Couscous, cooked	1 cup	176	Tr	Tr	36	2.2	8	2 1/2	1/2 Starch
Flour, all-purpose, enriched	3 Tbsp	85	0.2	0	18	0.6	0.5	1	1 Starch
Flour, dry	3 Tbsp	80	0	0	15	0.6	0.5	1	1 Starch
Flour, self-rising, enriched	3 Tbsp	83	0.2	0	17	0.6	298	1	1 Starch
Flour, whole-wheat	3 Tbsp	76	0.4	0	16	2.8	1.1	1	1 Starch
Hominy, cooked	1 cup	145	Tr	0.1	31	0.5	0	2	2 Starch
Kasha, cooked (buckwheat groats)	1 cup	155	1	0.2	33	4.5	7	2	2 Starch
Millet, cooked	1 cup	207	1.7	0.3	41.2	2.3	3	3	2 1/2 Starch
Muesli	1/2 cup	144	2.3	0.4	31.3	2.8	53	2	2 Starch
Plantain Flour, commercial	3 Tbsp	71	0.2	0	19	0.3	0	1	1 Starch
Poi	1 cup	269	0.3	0.1	65.4	1	29	4	4 Starch
Polenta	1/2 cup	320	0	0	72	8	0	5	4 Starch
Quinoa, dry	1/2 cup	318	4.9	0.5	58.6	5	18	4	4 Starch
Rice									
Basmati, cooked	1 cup	205	0.4	0.1	44.5	0.6	604	3	3 Starch

	Portion	Cal	Fat (g)	Sat Fat (g)	Carb (g)	Fiber (g)	Sod (mgs)	Carb Choices	Exchanges
Brown, long-grain, cooked	1 cup	216	2	0.4	45	3.5	10	3	3 Starch
Fried	1 cup	271	12	1.8	34	1.3	261	2	2 Starch,2 Fat
Instant, prepared	1 cup	162	Tr	0.1	35	1	5	3	2 Starch
White, long-grain, cooked	1 cup	205	Tr	0.1	45	0.6	2	3	3 Starch
Wild, cooked	1 cup	166	1	0.1	35	3	5	2	2 Starch
Tempeh	1 cup	320	18	3.7	15	9	15	1	2 Starch, 3 Lean Meat
Wheat germ, toasted, plain	1 Tbsp	27	1	0.1	3	0.9	Tr	0	1/3 Starch
Yam, yam pie									
Fresh root, raw	1/2 cup	89	0.1	0	21	0	7	1 1/2	1 1/2 Starch
Fresh root, cooked	1 small	95	0	0	21	0	7	1 1/2	1 1/2 Starch
Flour	3 Tbsp	74	0	0	18	0.4	0	1	1 Starch
Noodles/Pasta									
Cellophane, dehydrated	1 cup	491	0.1	<0.1	120.5	0.7	14	8	8 Starch
Chow mein, canned	1 cup	237	14	2	26	1.8	198	2	2 Starch
Egg noodles, cooked	1 cup	213	2	0.5	40	1.8	11	2 1/2	3 Starch

	Portion	Cal	Fat (g)	Sat Fat (g)	Carb (g)	Fiber (g)	Sod (mgs)	Carb Choices	Exchanges
Elbow macaroni, enriched, cooked	1 cup	197	1	0.1	40	1.8	1	2 1/2	3 Starch
Pasta, cooked	1/2 cup	95	0.5	0	19	0.9	1	1	1 1/4 Starch
Ramen, cooked	1 cup	154	6.5	1.7	20.2	1.2	802	1	1 1/2 Starch, 1 Fat
Ramen, low-fat	1 cup	110	0.8	0.5	22.5	1	650	1 1/2	1 1/2 Starch
Spaghetti, cooked, enriched	1 cup	197	1	0.1	40	2.4	1	2 1/2	2 1/2 Starch
Spaghetti, whole-wheat, cooked	1 cup	174	1	0.1	37	6.3	4	2 1/2	2 1/2 Starch
Udon, cooked	1/2 cup	115	0.6	0	23	0.1	51	1 1/2	1 1/2 Starch
Starchy Vegetables									
Corn									
On cob, from raw, cooked	1 ear	83	1	0.2	19	2.2	13	1	1 Starch
On cob, frozen, cooked	1 ear	59	Tr	0.1	14	1.8	3	1	1 Starch
Kernels, from frozen, cooked	1 cup	131	1	0.1	32	3.9	8	2	2 Starch
Cream style, canned	1 cup	184	1	0.2	46	3.1	730	3	3 Starch
Vacuum-packed	1 cup	166	1	0.2	41	4.2	571	3	2 1/2 Starch

	Portion	Cal	Fat (g)	Sat Fat (g)	Carb (g)	Fiber (g)	Sod (mgs)	Carb Choices	Exchanges
Eddo, dasheen, taro									
Fresh tuber, raw	1/2 cup	58	0.1	0	13.8	2.1	6	1	1 Starch
Tuber, cooked	1/2 cup	94	0	0	22.8	3.4	10	1 1/2	1/2 Starch
Tuber, fried	½ cup	164	5.7	1.5	27.7	4	198	2	2 Starch, 1 Fat
Malanga, cooked	1 cup	188	0.4	0.1	47	7.2	427	3	3 Starch
Parsnips, cooked	1 cup	126	Tr	0.1	30	6.2	16	2	2 Starch
Plantain, cooked slices	1 cup	179	Tr	0.1	48	3.5	8	3	3 Starch
Potatoes									
Au gratin, homemade	1 cup	323	19	11.6	28	4.4	1,061	2	2 Starch, 4 Fat
Au gratin, prepared from mix	1 cup	228	10	6.3	31	2.2	1,076	2	2 Starch, 2 Fat
Baked, with skin	1 potato	220	Tr	0.1	51	4.8	16	3 1/2	3 1/2 Starch
Baked, without skin	1 potato	145	Tr	Tr	34	2.3	8	2	2 Starch
Boiled	1 cup	134	Tr	Tr	31	2.8	8	2	2 Starch
French-fried, oven-heated	10 strips	100	4	0.6	16	1.6	15	1	1 Starch, 1 Fat
French-fried, restaurant	20–25 fries	458	24.7	5.2	53.3	4.7	265	3 1/2	3 1/2 Starch, 5 Fat
Hash browns, frozen	1 patty	63	3	1.3	8	0.6	10	1/2	1/2 Starch, 1/2 Fat

	Portion	Cal	Fat (g)	Sat Fat (g)	Carb (g)	Fiber (g)	Sod (mgs)	Carb Choices	Exchanges
Hash browns, homemade	1 cup	326	22	8.5	33	3.1	37	2	2 Starch, 4 Fat
Mashed, homemade	1 cup	237	12	7.2	32	4.8	697	2	2 Starch, 2 1/2 Fat
Mashed, from mix	1 cup	223	9	2.2	35	4.2	620	2	2 Starch, 2 Fat
Sweet potato, baked with skin	1 potato	150	Tr	Tr	35	4.4	15	2	2 Starch
Sweet potato, boiled, no skin	1 potato	164	Tr	0.1	38	2.8	20	2 1/2	2 1/2 Starch
Sweet potato, candied	21/2"×2" pc	144	3	1.4	29	2.5	74	2	2 Starch
Sweet potato, canned in syrup	1 cup	212	1	0.1	50	5.9	76	3	4 Starch
Squash									
Winter, all varieties, baked	1 cup	80	1	0.3	18	5.7	2	1	1 1/2 Starch
Winter, butternut, frozen, cooked	1 cup	94	Tr	Tr	24	2.2	5	1 1/2	1 1/2 Starch

Chapter 16

Fruit Choices

Any fruit or 100% fruit juice counts as part of the fruit group. Fruits may be fresh, canned, frozen, or dried, and may be whole, cut-up, or pureed.

A diet rich in potassium may help to maintain healthy blood pressure. Prune juice, bananas, cantaloupe, honeydew, prunes, dried peaches or apricots, orange juice, and plantains are all rich in potassium.

The Dietary Guidelines suggest you eat 2 cups of fruit every day.

Fruit Tips:

- Eat fruits raw, as juice with no sugar added, or canned in their own juice.

- Eat pieces of fruit, rather than drinking fruit juice. Pieces of fruit are more filling.

- Buy fruit juice that is 100% juice, with no added sugar.

- To increase fiber intake, choose whole or cut-up fruits more often as snacks or with meals, instead of juice.

FRUIT CHOICES

	Portion	Cal	Fat (g)	Sat Fat (g)	Carb (g)	Fiber (g)	Sod (mgs)	Carb Choices	Exchanges
Ackee, fruit, raw	1/2 cup	180	17.5	0	5.5	.3	Tr	1/2	3 fat, 1/2 fruit
Apple, raw, whole	1 medium	81	Tr	0.1	21	3.7	0	1 1/2	1 1/2 Fruit
Apple, raw, peeled and sliced	1 cup	63	Tr	0.1	16	2.1	0	1	1 Fruit
Apple, dried	5 rings	78	Tr	Tr	21	2.8	28	1 1/2	1 1/2 Fruit
Apple juice	1 cup	117	Tr	Tr	29	0.2	7	2	2 Fruit
Applesauce, sweetened	1 cup	194	Tr	0.1	51	3.1	8	3 1/2	3 Fruit
Applesauce, unsweetened	1 cup	105	Tr	Tr	28	2.9	5	2	2 Fruit
Apricot, raw, no pit	1 apricot	17	Tr	Tr	4	0.8	Tr	0	1/4 Fruit
Apricot, canned, heavy syrup	1 cup	214	1	Tr	55	4.1	10	3 1/2	2 Fruit
Apricot, canned, juice-packed	1 cup	117	Tr	Tr	30	3.9	10	2	2 Fruit
Apricot, dried	10 halves	83	Tr	Tr	22	3.2	4	1 1/2	1 1/2 Fruit
Apricot nectar, canned	1 cup	141	Tr	Tr	36	1.5	8	2 1/2	2 Fruit
Asian pear, raw	1 small	51	Tr	Tr	13	4.4	0	1	1 Fruit
Banana, raw, whole	1 medium	109	1	0.2	28	2.8	1	2	2 Fruit
Banana, raw, sliced	1 cup	138	1	0.3	35	3.6	2	2	2 Fruit

	Portion	Cal	Fat (g)	Sat Fat (g)	Carb (g)	Fiber (g)	Sod (mgs)	Carb Choices	Exchanges
Blackberry, raw	1 cup	75	1	Tr	18	7.6	0	1	1 1/3 Fruit
Blueberry, raw	1 cup	81	1	Tr	20	3.9	9	1	1 1/3 Fruit
Blueberry, frozen, sweetened	1 cup	186	Tr	Tr	50	4.8	2	3	3 1/3 Fruit
Breadfruit	1 cup	227	0.51	0.10	60	10.8	4	4	4 Fruit
Cantaloupe, raw, wedge	1/8 melon	24	Tr	Tr	6	0.6	6	1/2	1/2 Fruit
Cantaloupe, raw, cubes	1 cup	56	Tr	0.1	13	1.3	14	1	1 Fruit
Carambola (starfruit), raw, whole	1 (3 5/8")	30	Tr	Tr	7	2.5	2	1/2	1/2 Fruit
Carambola (starfruit), raw, sliced	1 cup	36	Tr	Tr	8	2.9	2	1/2	1/2 Fruit
Cherry, sour, red, water-packed	1 cup	88	Tr	0.1	22	2.7	17	1 1/2	1 1/2 Fruit
Cherry, sweet, raw	10 cherries	49	1	0.1	11	1.6	0	1	1 Fruit
Cherry, West Indies									
Fruit, ripe	3 oz	32	0.3	0	7.7	0.4	7	1/2	1/2 Fruit
Juice, fresh	1/3 cup	21	0.3	0	4.8	0.3	3	0	1/3 Fruit
Chocho, christophine, chayote									
Fruit, raw	1 each	38	0.3	0	9	3.5	4	1/2	1 Fruit
Fruit, cooked, drained	1/2 cup	19	0.4	0	4	2.2	1	0	1/3 Fruit

	Portion	Cal	Fat (g)	Sat Fat (g)	Carb (g)	Fiber (g)	Sod (mgs)	Carb Choices	Exchanges
Cranberry, dried, sweetened	1/4 cup	92	Tr	Tr	24	2.5	1	1 1/2	1 1/2 Fruit
Cranberry sauce, sweetened, canned	1 slice	86	Tr	Tr	22	0.6	17	1 1/2	1 1/2 Fruit
Custard apple	1/2 cup	114	0.7	0.3	28	2.7	5	2	2 Fruit
Date, whole	5 dates	116	Tr	0.1	31	3.2	1	2	2 Fruit
Date, chopped	1 cup	490	1	0.3	131	13.4	5	9	8 Fruit
Fig, dried	2 figs	97	Tr	0.1	25	4.6	4	11/2	1 Fruit
Fruit cocktail, canned, heavy syrup	1 cup	181	Tr	Tr	47	2.5	15	3	3 Fruit
Fruit cocktail, canned, juice-packed	1 cup	109	Tr	Tr	28	2.4	9	2	2 Fruit
Governor plum	3 oz	108	0	0	29.5	0.5	0	2	2 Fruit
Grapefruit, raw, pink or red	1/2 fruit	37	Tr	Tr	9	1.4	0	1/2	1 Fruit
Grapefruit, raw, white	1/2 fruit	39	Tr	Tr	10	1.3	0	1/2	1 Fruit
Grapefruit, canned, light syrup	1 cup	152	Tr	Tr	39	1	5	2 1/2	2 1/3 Fruit
Grapefruit juice, raw, pink	1 cup	96	Tr	Tr	23	0.2	2	1 1/2	2 Fruit
Grapefruit juice, raw, white	1 cup	96	Tr	Tr	23	0.2	2	1 1/2	2 Fruit

	Portion	Cal	Fat (g)	Sat Fat (g)	Carb (g)	Fiber (g)	Sod (mgs)	Carb Choices	Exchanges
Grapefruit juice, canned, unsweetened	1 cup	94	Tr	Tr	22	0.2	2	1 1/2	2 Fruit
Grapefruit juice, canned, sweetened	1 cup	115	Tr	Tr	28	0.3	5	2	2 Fruit
Grapefruit juice, frozen conc., dilute	1 cup	101	Tr	Tr	24	0.2	2	1 1/2	2 Fruit
Grape, seedless, raw	10 grapes	36	Tr	0.1	9	0.5	1	1/2	1/2 Fruit
Grape juice, canned or bottled	1 cup	154	Tr	0.1	38	0.3	8	2 1/2	3 Fruit
Grape juice, frzn conc, swtned, dilute	1 cup	128	Tr	0.1	32	0.3	5	2	2 Fruit
Guava									
Raw	1 cup	112	2	0	24	9	3	1 1/2	2 Fruit
Pulp only	1/2 cup	42	0.5	0.1	9.8	4.5	2	1/2	1 Fruit
Nectar	4 fld ounces	72	0.1	0	18	1.8	0	1	1 1/4 Fruit
Guinep, genip	3 oz	59	0.2	0	19.9	1.4	0	1	1 1/4 Fruit
Hog plum	3 oz	70	2.1	0	13.8	1	0	1	1 Fruit
Honeydew, wedge	1/8 melon	56	Tr	Tr	15	1	16	1	1 Fruit
Honeydew, diced	1 cup	60	Tr	Tr	16	1	17	1	1 Fruit
Jackfruit	1/2 cup	78	0.3	0	19.8	1.3	2	1	1 1/3 Fruit
Java plum	1 cup	81	0	0	21	0	19	1 1/2	1 1/2 Fruit
Jujube	3 oz	79	0.2	0	20.2	1.4	3	1	1 Fruit

	Portion	Cal	Fat (g)	Sat Fat (g)	Carb (g)	Fiber (g)	Sod (mgs)	Carb Choices	Exchanges
Kiwi fruit, raw, without skin	1 medium	46	Tr	Tr	11	2.6	4	1	1 Fruit
Lemon, raw, no peel	1 (2 1/8")	17	Tr	Tr	5	1.6	1	0	Free Food
Lemon juice, raw	1 lemon	12	0	0	4	0.2	Tr	0	Free Food
Lemon juice, bottled, unsweetened	1 Tbsp	3	Tr	Tr	1	0.1	3	0	Free Food
Lime juice, raw	1 lime	10	Tr	Tr	3	0.2	Tr	0	Free Food
Lime juice, canned, unsweetened	1 Tbsp	3	Tr	Tr	1	0.1	2	0	Free Food
Mamey apple	1/4	108	1	0	27	6	32	2	2 Fruit
Mango, raw, whole	1 mango	135	1	0.1	35	3.7	4	2	2 Fruit
Mango, raw, sliced	1 cup	107	Tr	0.1	28	3	3	2	2 Fruit
Mangosteen, canned, drained	1/2 cup	76	0.8	0	18.6	1.3	0	1	1 Fruit
Muskmelon	4 oz	40	0.3	0	9.4	0.9	10	1/2	1 Fruit
Nectarine, raw	1 small	67	1	0.1	16	2.2	0	1	1 Fruit
Orange, raw, whole	1 small	62	Tr	Tr	15	3.1	0	1	1 Fruit
Orange, raw, sections	1 cup	85	Tr	Tr	21	4.3	0	1 1/2	1 1/2 Fruit
Orange juice, raw	1 cup	112	Tr	0.1	26	0.5	2	2	2 Fruit

	Portion	Cal	Fat (g)	Sat Fat (g)	Carb (g)	Fiber (g)	Sod (mgs)	Carb Choices	Exchanges
Orange juice, canned, unsweetened	1 cup	105	Tr	Tr	25	0.5	5	1 1/2	2 Fruit
Orange juice, chilled, refrigerated	1 cup	110	1	0.1	25	0.5	2	1 1/2	2 Fruit
Orange juice, frozen conc, diluted	1 cup	112	Tr	0.1	27	0.5	2	2	2 Fruit
Papaya, raw, 1/2" cubes	1 cup	55	Tr	0.1	14	2.5	4	1	1 Fruit
Papaya, raw, whole	1 papaya	119	Tr	0.1	30	5.5	9	2	2 Fruit
Passion fruit/ granadilla	1/2 cup	114	0.8	0	27.6	12	33	2	2 Fruit
Pawpaw, papaya									
Fresh fruit	1/2 medium	59	0.2	0	14.9	2.7	5	1	1 Fruit
Nectar, canned	4 fld ounces	71	0.2	0	18	0.8	6	1	1 1/3 Fruit
Peach, raw, whole	1 (2 1/2")	42	Tr	Tr	11	2	0	1	1 Fruit
Peach, canned, heavy syrup	1 half	73	Tr	Tr	20	1.3	6	1	1 Fruit
Peach, canned, juice-packed	1 half	43	Tr	Tr	11	1.3	4	1	1 Fruit
Peach, dried, sulfured	3 halves	93	Tr	Tr	24	3.2	3	1 1/2	1 1/2 Fruit
Peach, frozen, sweetened	1 cup	235	Tr	Tr	60	4.5	15	4	4 Fruit

	Portion	Cal	Fat (g)	Sat Fat (g)	Carb (g)	Fiber (g)	Sod (mgs)	Carb Choices	Exchanges
Pear, raw, with skin	1 (2 1/2")	98	1	Tr	25	4	0	1 1/2	1 1/2 Fruit
Pear, canned, heavy syrup	1 half	56	Tr	Tr	15	1.2	4	1	1 Fruit
Pear, canned, juice-packed	1 half	38	Tr	Tr	10	1.2	3	1/2	1/2 Fruit
Pineapple, raw, diced	1 cup	76	1	Tr	19	1.9	2	1	1 1/4 Fruit
Pineapple, canned, heavy syrup	1 cup	198	Tr	Tr	51	2	3	3 1/2	3 Fruit
Pineapple, canned, heavy syrup	1 slice	38	Tr	Tr	10	0.4	Tr	1/2	1/2 Fruit
Pineapple, canned, juice-packed	1 cup	149	Tr	Tr	39	2	2	2 1/2	2 Fruit
Pineapple, canned, juice-packed	1 slice	28	Tr	Tr	7	0.4	Tr	1/2	1/2 Fruit
Pineapple, canned, unsweetened	1 cup	140	Tr	Tr	34	0.5	3	2	2 Fruit
Plantain, raw, without peel	1 medium	218	1	0.3	57	4.1	7	4	3 Fruit
Plantain, cooked, slices	1 cup	179	Tr	0.1	48	3.5	8	3	2 Fruit
Plum, raw	1 (2 1/8")	36	Tr	Tr	9	1	0	1/2	1/2 Fruit
Plum, canned, heavy syrup	1 cup	230	Tr	Tr	60	2.6	49	4	4 Fruit

	Portion	Cal	Fat (g)	Sat Fat (g)	Carb (g)	Fiber (g)	Sod (mgs)	Carb Choices	Exchanges
Plum, canned, heavy syrup	1 plum	41	Tr	Tr	11	0.5	9	1	1 Fruit
Plum, canned, juice-packed	1 cup	146	Tr	Tr	38	2.5	3	2 1/2	2 Fruit
Plum, canned, juice-packed	1 plum	27	Tr	Tr	7	0.5	Tr	1/2	1/2 Fruit
Prickly pear, raw	1 cup	61	0.7	0	14	2.7	7	1	1 Fruit
Prune, dried, pitted, uncooked	5 prunes	100	Tr	Tr	26	3	2	2	2 Fruit
Prune, stewed, unsweetened	1 cup	265	1	Tr	70	16.4	5	4 1/2	4 1/2 Fruit
Prune juice, canned or bottled	1 cup	182	Tr	Tr	45	2.6	10	3	3 Fruit
Raisin, seedless	1 cup	435	1	0.2	115	5.8	17	7 1/2	8 Fruit
Raisin, seedless	1/2 oz pack	42	Tr	Tr	11	0.6	2	1	3/4 Fruit
Raspberry, raw	1 cup	60	1	Tr	14	8.4	0	1	1 Fruit
Raspberry, frozen, sweetened	1 cup	258	Tr	Tr	65	11	3	4	4 Fruit
Rhubarb, frozen, cooked w/sugar	1 cup	278	Tr	Tr	75	4.8	2	5	5 Fruit
Rose apple	3 oz	25	0.3	0	5.7	1.1	0	1/2	1/2 Fruit
Sapodilla, naseberry	1/2 cup	100	1.3	0.2	24	6.4	14	1 1/2	1 1/2 Fruit
Sorrel, raw	3 oz	55	1	0	12	1	0	1	1 Fruit
Sorrel, dried	1 oz	101	.86	0	25	4	0	1 1/2	1 1/2 Fruit

	Portion	Cal	Fat (g)	Sat Fat (g)	Carb (g)	Fiber (g)	Sod (mgs)	Carb Choices	Exchanges
Soursop	1/4 Fruit	103	0.5	0	26.3	5.1	22	2	1 3/4 Fruit
Strawberries, raw, medium	1 (1 1/4")	4	Tr	Tr	1	0.3	Tr	0	Free Food
Strawberries, raw, sliced	1 cup	50	1	Tr	12	3.8	2	1	1 Fruit
Strawberries, frozen, sweetened	1 cup	245	Tr	Tr	66	4.8	8	4 1/2	4 Fruit
Surinam cherry	1 cup	57	1	0	13	0	5	1	1 Fruit
Sweetsop, sugar apple	1 Fruit	145	0	0	37	7	14	2 1/2	2 1/2 Fruit
Tangerine, raw, peeled	1 (2 3/8")	37	Tr	Tr	9	1.9	1	1/2	1/2 Fruit
Tangerine, canned, light syrup	1 cup	154	Tr	Tr	41	1.8	15	3	3 Fruit
Tangerine juice, canned, sweetened	1 cup	125	Tr	Tr	30	0.5	2	2	2 Fruit
Watermelon, raw, wedge	1/16 melon	92	1	0.1	21	1.4	6	1 1/2	1 1/2 Fruit
Watermelon, raw, diced	1 cup	49	1	0.1	11	0.8	3	1	1 Fruit

Chapter 17

Vegetable Choices

Any vegetable or 100% vegetable juice counts as a member of the vegetable group. Fresh, frozen, and canned vegetables all count toward meeting vegetable intake goals. For canned vegetables, "no salt added" is the best choice.

A diet rich in potassium may help to maintain healthy blood pressure. The following vegetables are rich in potassium: sweet potatoes, beet greens, white potatoes, white beans, tomato products, soybeans, lima beans, winter squash, spinach, lentils, kidney beans, and split peas.

The Dietary Guidelines suggest you eat 2 1/2 cups of vegetables every day.

Vegetable Tips:

- Eat raw and cooked vegetables with little or no fat.

- Steam vegetables using a small amount of water or low-fat broth.

- Mix in some chopped onion or garlic.

- Use a little vinegar or some lemon or lime juice.

- Add a small piece of lean ham or smoked turkey.

- If you do use a small amount of fat, use canola, olive oil, or tub margarine instead of fat from meat, butter, or shortening.

VEGETABLE CHOICES

	Portion	Cal	Fat (g)	Sat Fat (g)	Carb (g)	Fiber (g)	Sod (mgs)	Carb Choices	Exchanges
Alfalfa, raw	1 cup	10	Tr	Tr	1	0.8	2	0	1/3 Veg
Artichoke, globe or French	1 cup	84	Tr	0.1	19	9.1	160	1	2 Veg
Artichoke, globe or French	1 medium	60	Tr	Tr	13	6.5	114	1	2 Veg
Asparagus, green, cooked from raw	1 cup	43	1	0.1	8	2.9	20	1/2	2 Veg
Asparagus, green, cooked from frozen	1 cup	50	1	0.2	9	2.9	7	1/2	2 Veg
Asparagus, green, canned, drained	1 cup	46	2	0.4	6	3.9	695	1/2	2 Veg
Bamboo shoots, canned, drained	1 cup	25	1	0.1	4	1.8	9	0	1 Veg
Beans									
Snap, cooked from raw, green	1 cup	44	Tr	0.1	10	4	4	1/2	2 Veg
Snap, cooked from raw, yellow	1 cup	44	Tr	0.1	10	4.1	4	1/2	2 Veg

	Portion	Cal	Fat (g)	Sat Fat (g)	Carb (g)	Fiber (g)	Sod (mgs)	Carb Choices	Exchanges
Snap, cooked from frozen, green	1 cup	38	Tr	0.1	9	4.1	12	1/2	2 Veg
Snap, cooked from frozen, yellow	1 cup	38	Tr	0.1	9	4.1	12	1/2	2 Veg
Snap, canned, drained, green	1 cup	27	Tr	Tr	6	2.6	354	1/2	1 Veg
Snap, canned, drained, yellow	1 cup	27	Tr	Tr	6	1.8	339	1/2	1 Veg
Bean sprouts (mung), raw	1 cup	31	Tr	Tr	6	1.9	6	1/2	1 Veg
Bean sprouts, cooked, drained	1 cup	26	Tr	Tr	5	1.5	12	1/2	1 Veg
Beet, cooked, drained, slices	1 cup	75	Tr	Tr	17	3.4	131	1	2 Veg
Beet, cooked, drained, whole	1 beet	22	Tr	Tr	5	1	39	0	1 Veg

	Portion	Cal	Fat (g)	Sat Fat (g)	Carb (g)	Fiber (g)	Sod (mgs)	Carb Choices	Exchanges
Beet, canned, drained, slices	1 cup	53	Tr	Tr	12	2.9	330	1	2 Veg
Beet, canned, drained, whole	1 beet	7	Tr	Tr	2	0.4	47	0	1/2 Veg
Beet greens, cooked, drained	1 cup	39	Tr	Tr	8	4.2	347	1/2	2 Veg
Broccoli, raw, chopped	1 cup	25	Tr	Tr	5	2.6	24	0	1 Veg
Broccoli, raw, spear	5" spear	9	Tr	Tr	2	0.9	8	0	1/2 Veg
Broccoli, cooked from raw	5" spear	10	Tr	Tr	2	1.1	10	0	1/2 Veg
Broccoli, frozen, cooked, chopped	1 cup	52	Tr	Tr	10	5.5	44	1/2	2 Veg
Brussels sprouts, cooked from raw	1 cup	61	1	0.2	14	4.1	33	1	2 Veg
Brussels sprouts, cooked from frozen	1 cup	65	1	0.1	13	6.4	36	1	2 Veg

	Portion	Cal	Fat (g)	Sat Fat (g)	Carb (g)	Fiber (g)	Sod (mgs)	Carb Choices	Exchanges
Cabbage, raw, shredded	1 cup	18	Tr	Tr	4	1.6	13	0	1 Veg
Cabbage, cooked, drained	1 cup	33	1	0.1	7	3.5	12	1/2	2 Veg
Cabbage, Chinese, bok choy, cooked	1 cup	20	Tr	Tr	3	2.7	58	0	1 Veg
Cabbage, Chinese, pak choi, cooked	1 cup	20	Tr	Tr	3	2.7	58	0	1 Veg
Cabbage, Chinese, pe tsai, cooked	1 cup	17	Tr	Tr	3	3.2	11	0	1 Veg
Cabbage, red, raw, shredded	1 cup	19	Tr	Tr	4	1.4	8	0	1 Veg
Cabbage, Savoy, raw, shredded	1 cup	19	Tr	Tr	4	2.2	20	0	1 Veg
Callaloo, cooked	1/2 cup	19	0.2	0	3.7	1.2	19	0	1/2 Veg
Carrot juice, canned	1 cup	94	Tr	0.1	22	1.9	68	1 1/2	4 Veg
Carrot, raw, whole, 7–1/2" long	1 whole	31	Tr	Tr	7	2.2	25	1/2	1 Veg
Carrot, raw, baby	1 medium	4	Tr	Tr	1	0.2	4	0	1/4 Veg

	Portion	Cal	Fat (g)	Sat Fat (g)	Carb (g)	Fiber (g)	Sod (mgs)	Carb Choices	Exchanges
Carrot, cooked, drained, from raw	1 cup	70	Tr	0.1	16	5.1	103	1	2 Veg
Carrot, cooked, drained, from frozen	1 cup	53	Tr	Tr	12	5.1	86	1	2 Veg
Carrot, canned, drained	1 cup	37	Tr	0.1	8	2.2	353	1/2	1 Veg
Cauliflower, raw	1 floweret	3	Tr	Tr	1	0.3	4	0	1/4 Veg
Cauliflower, raw	1 cup	25	Tr	Tr	5	2.5	30	0	1 Veg
Cauliflower, cooked, from raw	1 cup	29	1	0.1	5	3.3	19	0	1 Veg
Cauliflower, cooked, from frozen	1 cup	34	Tr	0.1	7	4.9	32	1/2	1 Veg
Celery, raw, stalk, 7 1/2–8"	1 stalk	6	Tr	Tr	1	0.7	35	0	1/4 Veg
Celery, raw, pieces, diced	1 cup	19	Tr	Tr	4	2	104	0	1 Veg
Chives, raw, chopped	1 tbsp	1	Tr	Tr	Tr	0.1	Tr	0	Free Food (Less than 5 g carb and 20 calories)

	Portion	Cal	Fat (g)	Sat Fat (g)	Carb (g)	Fiber (g)	Sod (mgs)	Carb Choices	Exchanges
Cilantro, raw	1 tsp	Tr	Tr	Tr	Tr	Tr	1	0	Free Food
Coleslaw, home-made	1 cup	83	3	0.5	15	1.8	28	1	3 Veg, 2 Fat
Collards, cooked, from raw	1 cup	49	1	0.1	9	5.3	17	1/2	2 Veg
Collards, cooked, from frozen	1 cup	61	1	0.1	12	4.8	85	1	2 Veg
Cucumber, peeled, sliced	1 cup	14	Tr	Tr	3	0.8	2	0	1 Veg
Cucumber, whole, peeled	1 large	34	Tr	0.1	7	2	6	1/2	1 1/2 Veg
Cucumber, unpeeled, sliced	1 cup	14	Tr	Tr	3	0.8	2	0	1 Veg
Cucumber, whole, unpeeled	1 large	39	Tr	0.1	8	2.4	6	1/2	1 1/2 Veg
Dandelion greens, cooked	1 cup	35	1	0.2	7	3	46	1/2	2 Veg
Dill weed, raw	5 sprigs	Tr	Tr	Tr	Tr	Tr	1	0	Free Food
Eggplant, cooked, drained	1 cup	28	Tr	Tr	7	2.5	3	1/2	2 Veg
Endive, curly, raw	1 cup	9	Tr	Tr	2	1.6	11	0	1 Veg
Garlic, raw	1 clove	4	Tr	Tr	1	0.1	1	0	1/4 Veg

	Portion	Cal	Fat (g)	Sat Fat (g)	Carb (g)	Fiber (g)	Sod (mgs)	Carb Choices	Exchanges
Hearts of palm, canned	1 piece	9	Tr	Tr	2	0.8	141	0	1/2 Veg
Jerusalem artichoke, raw	1 cup	114	Tr	0	26	2.4	6	2	1 Veg
Kale, cooked, from raw	1 cup	36	1	0.1	7	2.6	30	1/2	2 Veg
Kale, cooked, from frozen	1 cup	39	1	0.1	7	2.6	20	1/2	2 Veg
Kohlrabi, cooked, drained	1 cup	48	Tr	Tr	11	1.8	35	1	2 Veg
Leeks, bulb and lower leaf, cooked	1 cup	32	Tr	Tr	8	1	10	1/2	2 Veg
Lettuce, butterhead, raw, leaf	1 med leaf	1	Tr	Tr	Tr	0.1	Tr	0	Free Food
Lettuce, butterhead, raw, head	3 cups	21	Tr	Tr	4	1.6	8	0	1 Veg
Lettuce, crisphead, raw, leaf	1 medium	1	Tr	Tr	Tr	0.1	1	0	Free Food
Lettuce, crisphead, raw, head	1 head	65	1	0.1	11	7.5	49	1	2 1/2 Veg
Lettuce, crisphead, raw, pieces	1 cup	7	Tr	Tr	1	0.8	5	0	1 Veg

	Portion	Cal	Fat (g)	Sat Fat (g)	Carb (g)	Fiber (g)	Sod (mgs)	Carb Choices	Exchanges
Lettuce, looseleaf, leaf	1 leaf	2	Tr	Tr	Tr	0.2	1	0	Free Food
Lettuce, looseleaf, shredded	1 cup	10	Tr	Tr	2	1.1	5	0	1 Veg
Lettuce, romaine, inner leaf	1 leaf	1	Tr	Tr	Tr	0.2	1	0	Free Food
Lettuce, romaine, shredded	1 cup	8	Tr	Tr	1	1	4	0	1 Veg
Mushroom, raw, pieces	1 cup	18	Tr	Tr	3	0.8	3	0	1 Veg
Mushroom, cooked, drained	1 cup	42	1	0.1	8	3.4	3	1/2	2 Veg
Mushroom, canned, drained	1 cup	37	Tr	0.1	8	3.7	663	1/2	2 Veg
Mushroom, shitake, cooked	1 cup	80	Tr	0.1	21	3	6	1 1/2	2 Veg
Mushroom, shitake, dried	1 each	11	Tr	Tr	3	0.4	Tr	0	1/2 Veg
Mustard greens, cooked	1 cup	21	Tr	Tr	3	2.8	22	0	2 Veg
Okra, cooked from raw	1 cup	51	Tr	0.1	12	4	8	1	2 Veg

	Portion	Cal	Fat (g)	Sat Fat (g)	Carb (g)	Fiber (g)	Sod (mgs)	Carb Choices	Exchanges
Okra, cooked from frozen	1 cup	52	1	0.1	11	5.2	6	1	2 Veg
Onion, raw, chopped	1 cup	61	Tr	Tr	14	2.9	5	1	1 Veg
Onion, raw, whole	1 cup	42	Tr	Tr	9	2	3	1/2	1 Veg
Onion, raw, sliced	1 cup	5	Tr	Tr	1	0.3	Tr	0	1/4 Veg
Onion, cooked, drained	1 cup	92	Tr	0.1	21	2.9	6	1 1/2	2 Veg
Onion, dehydrated flakes	1 Tbsp	17	Tr	Tr	4	0.5	1	0	1/2 Veg
Onion, spring, raw, top and bulb	1 cup	32	Tr	Tr	7	2.6	16	1/2	1 Veg
Onion, spring, raw, top and bulb	1 whole	5	Tr	Tr	1	0.4	2	0	Free Food
Onion rings, breaded, frozen	10 rings	244	16	5.2	23	0.8	225	1 1/2	1 1/2 Starch, 3 Fat
Parsley, raw	10 sprigs	4	Tr	Tr	1	0.3	6	0	Free Food
Parsnip, cooked, drained	1 cup	126	Tr	0.1	30	6.2	16	2	2 Veg
Peppers									
Hot chili, raw, green or red	1 pepper	18	Tr	Tr	4	0.7	3	0	1 Veg

	Portion	Cal	Fat (g)	Sat Fat (g)	Carb (g)	Fiber (g)	Sod (mgs)	Carb Choices	Exchanges
Jalapeno, canned, solids and liquid	1/4 cup	7	Tr	Tr	1	0.7	434	0	1/3 Veg
Sweet, green, raw, chopped	1 cup	40	Tr	Tr	10	2.7	3	1/2	1 Veg
Sweet, green, raw, whole	1 pepper	32	Tr	Tr	8	2.1	2	1/2	1 Veg
Sweet, red, raw, chopped	1 cup	40	Tr	Tr	10	3	3	1/2	1 Veg
Sweet, red, raw, whole	1 pepper	32	Tr	Tr	8	2.4	2	1/2	1 Veg
Sweet, green or red, cooked	1 cup	38	Tr	Tr	9	1.6	3	1/2	2 Veg
Pimento, canned	1 Tbsp	3	Tr	Tr	1	0.2	2	0	Free Food
Radish, raw	1 radish	1	Tr	Tr	Tr	0.1	1	0	Free Food
Sauerkraut, canned, solids and liquid	1 cup	45	Tr	0.1	10	5.9	1560	1/2	2 Veg
Seaweed, kelp, raw	2 Tbsp	4	Tr	Tr	1	0.1	23	0	Free Food

	Portion	Cal	Fat (g)	Sat Fat (g)	Carb (g)	Fiber (g)	Sod (mgs)	Carb Choices	Exchanges
Seaweed, spirulina, dried	1 Tbsp	3	Tr	Tr	Tr	Tr	10	0	Free Food
Shallots, raw, chopped	1 Tbsp	7	Tr	Tr	2	0.2	1	0	Free Food
Spinach, raw, chopped	1 cup	7	Tr	Tr	1	0.8	24	0	1 Veg
Spinach, cooked from raw	1 cup	41	Tr	0.1	7	4.3	126	1/2	2 Veg
Spinach, cooked from frozen	1 cup	53	Tr	0.1	10	5.7	163	1/2	2 Veg
Spinach, canned	1 cup	49	1	0.2	7	5.1	58	1/2	2 Veg
Squash, summer, raw	1 cup	23	Tr	Tr	5	2.1	2	0	1 Veg
Squash, summer, cooked	1 cup	36	1	0.1	8	2.5	2	1/2	2 Veg
Tomatillo, raw	1 medium	11	Tr	Tr	2	0.6	Tr	0	1/2 Veg
Tomato, raw									
Chopped or sliced	1 cup	38	1	0.1	8	2	16	1/2	1 Veg
Sliced, 1/4" thick	1 slice	4	Tr	Tr	1	0.2	2	0	Free Food
Whole, cherry	1 cherry	4	Tr	Tr	1	0.2	2	0	Free Food

	Portion	Cal	Fat (g)	Sat Fat (g)	Carb (g)	Fiber (g)	Sod (mgs)	Carb Choices	Exchanges
Whole, medium	1 each	26	Tr	0.1	6	1.4	11	1/2	1 Veg
Tomato									
Canned, solids and liquid	1 cup	46	Tr	Tr	10	2.4	355	1/2	2 Veg
Sun-dried, plain	1 piece	5	Tr	Tr	1	0.2	42	0	Free Food
Sun-dried, packed in oil	1 piece	6	Tr	0.1	1	0.2	8	0	Free Food
Tomato juice, canned, salt added	1 cup	41	Tr	Tr	10	1	877	1/2	2 Veg
Tomato products, canned									
Paste	1 cup	215	1	0.2	51	10.7	231	3 1/2	10 Veg
Puree	1 cup	100	Tr	0.1	24	5	85	1 1/2	4 Veg
Sauce	1 cup	74	Tr	0.1	18	3.4	1482	1	3 Veg
Stewed	1 cup	71	Tr	Tr	17	2.6	564	1	2 Veg
Turnip, cooked	1 cup	33	Tr	Tr	8	3.1	78	1/2	2 Veg
Turnip greens, cooked from raw	1 cup	29	Tr	0.1	6	5	42	1/2	2 Veg
Turnip greens, cooked from frozen	1 cup	49	1	0.2	8	5.6	25	1/2	2 Veg

	Portion	Cal	Fat (g)	Sat Fat (g)	Carb (g)	Fiber (g)	Sod (mgs)	Carb Choices	Exchanges
Vegetable juice cocktail, canned	1 cup	46	Tr	Tr	11	1.9	653	1	2 Veg
Vegetables, mixed, canned	1 cup	77	Tr	0.1	15	4.9	243	1	2 Veg
Vegetables, mixed, frozen	1 cup	107	Tr	0.1	24	8	64	1 1/2	2 Veg
Water chestnuts, canned	1 cup	70	Tr	Tr	17	3.5	11	1	1 Veg
Watercress	2 cups	7	0	0	0.8	0.3	28	0	Free Food

Chapter 18

Milk Choices

All fluid milk products and many foods made from milk are considered part of this food group. Although cheese is made from milk, it does not contain carbohydrate. Nutritionally, cheese is closer to meat. You can find cheese in the fish, poultry, and meat choices in Chapter 19.

If you don't or can't drink milk, choose lactose-free products or other calcium sources, such as fortified foods and beverages. Other sources of calcium include calcium-fortified beverages, fortified breakfast cereals, sardines, or tofu made with calcium if milk and milk products are not consumed.

The Dietary Guidelines suggest you drink 3 cups of milk every day.

Milk Tips:

- Choose fat-free (skim) or low-fat (1%) milk, yogurt, and cheese.
- Eat low-fat or fat-free yogurt, and choose calcium-fortified frozen yogurt or ice milk.

MILK CHOICES

	Portion	Cal	Fat (g)	Sat Fat (g)	Carb (g)	Fiber (g)	Sod (mgs)	Carb Choices	Exchanges
Milk, fluid, no milk solids added									
Whole (3.3% fat)	1 cup	150	8	5.1	11	0	120	1	1 Milk, 1 1/2 Fat
Reduced-fat (2%)	1 cup	121	5	2.9	12	0	122	1	1 Milk, 1 Fat
Low-fat (1%)	1 cup	102	3	1.6	12	0	123	1	1 Milk, 1/2 Fat
Non-fat (skim)	1 cup	86	Tr	0.3	12	0	126	1	1 Milk
Buttermilk	1 cup	99	2	1.3	12	0	257	1	1 Milk
Canned Milk									
Condensed, sweetened	1 cup	982	27	16.8	166	0	389	11	11 Starch, 5 Fat
Evaporated, whole	1 cup	339	19	11.6	25	0	267	1 1/2	2 Milk, 4 Fat
Evaporated, skim	1 cup	199	1	0.3	29	0	294	2	2 Milk
Dried Milk									
Buttermilk	1 cup	464	7	4.3	59	0	621	4	4 Milk, 1 1/2 Fat
Non-fat, instant, Vit. A added	1 cup	244	Tr	0.3	35	0	373	2	2 Milk
Milk Beverages									
Chocolate milk, whole	1 cup	208	8	5.3	26	2	149	2	2 Starch, 1 1/2 Fat

	Portion	Cal	Fat (g)	Sat Fat (g)	Carb (g)	Fiber (g)	Sod (mgs)	Carb Choices	Exchanges
Chocolate milk, reduced-fat (2%)	1 cup	179	5	3.1	26	1.3	151	2	2 Starch, 1 Fat
Chocolate milk, low-fat (1%)	1 cup	158	3	1.5	26	1.3	152	2	2 Starch, 1/2 Fat
Eggnog (commercial)	1 cup	342	19	11.3	34	0	138	2	2 Starch, 4 Fat
Milk shake, thick, chocolate	10.6 fl oz	356	8	5	63	0.9	333	4	4 Starch, 2 Fat
Milk shake, thick, vanilla	11 fl oz	350	9	5.9	56	0	299	4	4 Starch, 2 Fat
Frozen yogurt, soft serve									
Chocolate	1/2 cup	115	4	2.6	18	1.6	71	1	1 Starch, 1 Fat
Vanilla	1/2 cup	114	4	2.5	17	0	63	1	1 Starch, 1 Fat
Ice cream									
Chocolate, regular	1/2 cup	143	7	4.5	19	0.8	50	1	1 Starch, 2 Fats
Vanilla, regular	1/2 cup	133	7	4.5	16	0	53	1	1 Starch, 2 Fats
Vanilla, light (50% reduced fat)	1/2 cup	92	3	1.7	15	0	56	1	1 Starch, 1 Fat
Chocolate, low-fat	1/2 cup	113	2	1	22	0.7	50	1 1/2	1 Starch, 1 Fat
Vanilla, rich	1/2 cup	178	12	7.4	17	0	41	1	1 Starch, 2 Fats

	Portion	Cal	Fat (g)	Sat Fat (g)	Carb (g)	Fiber (g)	Sod (mgs)	Carb Choices	Exchanges
Vanilla, soft serve	1/2 cup	185	11	6.4	19	0	52	1	1 Starch, 2 Fats
Sherbet	1/2 cup	102	1	0.9	22	0	34	1 1/2	2 Starch
Yogurt									
Fruit-flavored, low-fat	8 oz	231	2	1.6	43	0	133	3	3 Starch
Plain, low-fat	8 oz	144	4	2.3	16	0	159	1	1 Milk, 1 Fat
Fruit-flavored, non-fat	8 oz	213	Tr	0.3	43	0	132	3	3 Starch
Plain, non-fat	8 oz	127	Tr	0.3	17	0	174	1	1 Starch
Plain, whole milk	8 oz	139	7	4.8	11	0	105	1	1 Starch, 1 1/2 Fat
Vanilla, non-fat, lo-cal, sweetener	8 oz	98	Tr	0.3	17	0	134	1	1 Milk
Lemon, non-fat, lo-cal, sweetener	8 oz	98	Tr	0.3	17	0	134	1	1 Milk
Other Milk									
Buffalo's milk, whole	8 fluid oz	237	17	11.2	12.7	0	127	1	1 milk, 2 fat
Goat's milk, whole	8 fluid oz	168	10	6.6	11	0	122	1	1 milk, 1 fat
Sheep's milk, whole	8 fluid oz	264	17	11.2	13	0	107	1	1 milk, 2 fat
Human milk	8 fluid oz	171	11	4.8	16.8	0	41.5	1	1 milk, 1 fat

Chapter 19

Fish, Poultry, and Meat Choices

All foods made from meat, poultry, and fish are part of this group. Nutritionally, cheese is closer to meat and can be found in this group. Choose fat-free or low fat cheese. Most meat and poultry choices should be lean or low-fat. Fish contain healthy oils, so choose these foods frequently instead of meat or poultry. Processed meats, such as ham, sausage, frankfurters, and luncheon or deli meats, have added sodium. Fresh chicken, turkey, and pork that have been enhanced with a solution containing salt also have added sodium. Look on the label for statements like "self-basting," which mean that a solution containing sodium has been added to the product.

The Dietary Guidelines suggest you eat 5 1/2 oz of fish, poultry, or meat every day.

Fish, Poultry, and Meat Tips:

- Buy cuts of beef, pork, ham, and lamb that have only a little fat on them.

- Buy ground beef that is at least 90% lean.

- Eat chicken or turkey without the skin.

- Use cooking methods that do not add fat, such as grilling, broiling, poaching, or roasting.

- Choose lean turkey, roast beef, or ham or low-fat luncheon meats for sandwiches instead of fatty luncheon meats, such as regular bologna or salami.

- Choose fish rich in omega-3 fatty acids, such as salmon, trout, and herring.

FISH, POULTRY, and MEAT CHOICES

	Portion	Cal	Fat (g)	Sat Fat (g)	Carb (g)	Fiber (g)	Sod (mgs)	Carb Choices	Exchanges
Amberjack									
Raw	1 oz	24	0.3	0	0	0	0	0	1 Very Lean Meat
Dried	1 oz	76	1.3	0	0	0	0	0	1 Very Lean Meat
Anchovy	1 oz	24	0.3	0	0	0	0	0	1 Very Lean Meat
Barracuda	1 oz	31	0.7	0	0	0	0	0	1 Very Lean Meat
Bonito	1 oz	47	2	0	0	0	0	0	1 Very Lean Meat
Butterfish									
Raw	1 oz	41	2.2	0	0	0	25	0	1 Very Lean Meat
Baked	1 oz	52	2.9	0	0	0	32	0	1 Very Lean Meat
Carp, common	1 oz	35	1.6	0.3	0	0	14	0	1 Very Lean Meat
Catfish, breaded, fried	1 oz	65	4	1	2	0.2	79	0	1 Medium-Fat Meat
Clam, raw, meat only	1 oz	21	Tr	Tr	0.7	0	16	0	1 Very Lean Meat
Clam, raw, meat only	1 medium	11	Tr	Tr	Tr	0	3	0	1/2 Very Lean Meat
Clam, breaded, fried	3/4 cup	451	26	6.6	39	0.3	834	2.5	3 Medium-Fat Meat
Clam, canned, drained solids	1 oz	42	0.7	Tr	1	0	32	0	1 Very Lean Meat
Cod, baked or broiled	1 oz	30	Tr	Tr	0	0	26	0	1 Very Lean Meat

	Portion	Cal	Fat (g)	Sat Fat (g)	Carb (g)	Fiber (g)	Sod (mgs)	Carb Choices	Exchanges
Cod, baked or broiled	1 fillet	95	1	0.1	0	0	82	0	3 Very Lean Meat
Codfish, dehydrated, salted	1 oz	104	0.8	0	0	0	2250	0	1 Very Lean Meat
Crab, Alaska King, steamed	1 leg	130	2	0.2	0	0	1436	0	4 1/2 Very Lean Meat
Crab, Alaska King, steamed	1 oz	27	Tr	Tr	0	0	304	0	1 Very Lean Meat
Crab, imitation from surimi	1 oz	29	Tr	Tr	3	0	238	0	1 Very Lean Meat
Crab, blue, steamed	1 oz	29	0.7	Tr	0	0	79	0	1 Very Lean Meat
Crab, blue, canned crab meat	1 cup	134	2	0.3	0	0	450	0	4 1/2 Very Lean Meat
Crab cake, w/egg, onion, margarine	1 cake	93	5	0.9	Tr	0	198	0	2Very Lean Meat,1 Fat
Crawfish	1 oz	19	0.26	0.04	0	0	17	0	1 Very Lean Meat
Croaker, cooked	1 oz	37	0.9	0	0	0	33	0	1 Very Lean Meat
Croaker, raw	1 oz	29	0.9	0.3	0	0	24	0	1 Very Lean Meat
Dogfish	1 oz	43	2.5	0	0	0	0	0	1 Very Lean Meat
Dolphin	1 oz	24	0.2	0	0	0	24	0	1 Very Lean Meat
Eel, pike eel	1 oz	28	0.3	0	0	0	0	0	1 Very Lean Meat

	Portion	Cal	Fat (g)	Sat Fat (g)	Carb (g)	Fiber (g)	Sod (mgs)	Carb Choices	Exchanges
Fish fillet, battered/ breaded, fried	1 fillet	211	11	2.6	15	0.5	484	1	3 Medium-Fat Meat
Fish roe, cooked	1 oz	57	2.3	0.5	0.5	0	0	0	1 Lean Meat
Fish stick, breaded, frozen, reheated	1 stick	76	3	0.9	7	0	163	0.5	1/2 Lean Meat, 1/2 Fat, 1/2 Starch
Flounder or sole, baked or broiled	1 oz	33	Tr	Tr	0	0	30	0	1 Very Lean Meat
Frog legs	1 oz	20	0	0	0	0	0	0	1 Very Lean Meat
Flying fish	1 oz	25	0	0	0	0	0	0	1 Very Lean Meat
Haddock, baked or broiled	1 oz	32	Tr	Tr	0	0	25	0	1 Very Lean Meat
Halibut, baked or broiled	1 oz	40	0.7	Tr	0	0	20	0	1 Very Lean Meat
Herring, pickled	1 oz	74	5	0.7	3	0	247	0	1 Lean Meat
Herring, raw, whole	1 oz	54	3.9	0.9	0	0	21	0	1 Lean Meat
Jacks	1 oz	28	0.4	0	0	0	0	0	1 Very Lean Meat
Jewfish	1 oz	28	0.6	0	0	0	0	0	1 Very Lean Meat
Kingfish	1 oz	29	0.8	0	0	0	23	0	1 Very Lean Meat

	Portion	Cal	Fat (g)	Sat Fat (g)	Carb (g)	Fiber (g)	Sod (mgs)	Carb Choices	Exchanges
Lobster, steamed	1 oz	28	Tr	Tr	Tr	0	16	0	1 Very Lean Meat
Mackerel									
Raw	1 oz	62	4.5	0	0	0	36	0	1 Lean Meat
Canned, solids and liquids	1 oz	43	1.8	0.5	0	0	105	0	1 Very Lean Meat
Salted	1 oz	85	7	0	0	0	0	0	1 Medium-Fat Meat
Smoked	1 oz	61	3.6	0	0	0	0	0	1 Lean Meat
Mullet	1 oz	41	1.9	0	0	0	23	0	1 Very Lean Meat
Ocean perch, baked or broiled	1 oz	34	0.7	Tr	0	0	27	0	1 Very Lean Meat
Octopus	1 oz	46	0.6	0.1	1.2	0	0	0	1 Very Lean Meat
Oysters, raw, meat only	6 medium	57	2	0.6	3	0	177	0	1 Lean Meat
Oysters, breaded, fried	1 oz	56	4	1	3	Tr	118	0	1 Medium-Fat Meat
Parrot fish	1 oz	24	0.1	0	0	0	0	0	1 Very Lean Meat
Pollock, baked or broiled	1 oz	32	Tr	Tr	0	0	33	0	1 Very Lean Meat
Porgy	1 oz	31	0.9	0	0	0	0	0	1 Very Lean Meat
Rockfish, baked or broiled	1 oz	34	0.7	Tr	0	0	22	0	1 Very Lean Meat
Roughy, orange, baked or broiled	1 oz	25	Tr	Tr	0	0	23	0	1 Very Lean Meat

	Portion	Cal	Fat (g)	Sat Fat (g)	Carb (g)	Fiber (g)	Sod (mgs)	Carb Choices	Exchanges
Salmon, red, baked or broiled	1 oz	61	3	0.5	0	0	19	0	1 Lean Meat
Salmon, canned, solids and liquids	1 oz	39	2	Tr	0	0	157	0	1 Lean Meat
Sardines									
Raw	1 oz	44	2.4	0	0	0	0	0	1 Lean Meat
Canned, solids and liquids									
Canned in oil	1 oz	86	6.8	0.8	0.2	0	150	0	1 Medium-Fat Meat
Canned in tomato sauce	1 oz	55	3.4	0	0.5	0	111	0	1 Lean Meat
Scallops, breaded, fried	6 large	200	10	2.5	9	0.2	432	0	1 Medium-Fat Meat
Scallops, steamed	1 oz	32	Tr	Tr	1	0	75	0	1 Very Lean Meat
Sea bass	1 oz	22	0.1	0	0	0	0	0	1 Very Lean Meat
Shark	1 oz	18	0.6	0	0	0	0	0	1 Very Lean Meat
Shrimp, breaded, fried	1 oz	69	3	0.6	3	Tr	97	0	1 Medium-Fat Meat
Shrimp, canned, drained solids	1 oz	34	0.7	Tr	Tr	0	48	0	1 Very Lean Meat
Shrimp									
Raw	1 oz	24	0	0	0.7	0	39	0	1 Very Lean Meat
Dried, salted, shell eaten	1 oz	81	0.6	0	0.3	0	0	0	1 Very Lean Meat

	Portion	Cal	Fat (g)	Sat Fat (g)	Carb (g)	Fiber (g)	Sod (mgs)	Carb Choices	Exchanges
Snapper	1 oz	25	0.2	0	0	0	19	0	1 Very Lean Meat
Sole	1 oz	22	0.2	0	0	0	22	0	1 Very Lean Meat
Sturgeon									
Raw	1 oz	29	1.1	0.3	0	0	0	0	1 Very Lean Meat
Steamed	1 oz	26	0.1	0	0	0	0	0	1 Very Lean Meat
Swordfish, baked or broiled	1 oz	44	1	Tr	0	0	33	0	1 Very Lean Meat
Tilapia, raw	1 oz	29	0.8	0	0	0	0	0	1 Very Lean Meat
Trout, baked or broiled	1 oz	48	2	0.6	0	0	12	0	1 Very Lean Meat
Tuna, baked or broiled	1 oz	39	Tr	Tr	0	0	13	0	1 Very Lean Meat
Tuna, canned, oil-packed, chunk light	1 oz	56	2	0.5	0	0	100	0	1 Lean Meat
Tuna, canned, water-packed, chunk light	1 oz	33	Tr	Tr	0	0	96	0	1 Very Lean Meat
Tuna, canned, water-packed, solid white	1 oz	36	1	Tr	0	0	107	0	1 Very Lean Meat
Tuna salad	1 cup	383	19	3.2	19	0	824	1	4 Lean Meat,2 Fat,2 Starch
Turtle									
Raw	1 oz	25	0.1	0	0	0	0	0	1 Very Lean Meat

	Portion	Cal	Fat (g)	Sat Fat (g)	Carb (g)	Fiber (g)	Sod (mgs)	Carb Choices	Exchanges
Canned	1 oz	29	0.2	0	0	0	0	0	1 Very Lean Meat
Whiting, "Banga Mary"	1 oz	26	0.1	0	0	0	0	0	1 Very Lean Meat
Chicken									
Fried in vegetable oil, with skin									
Batter-dipped, breast	1/2 breast	364	18	4.9	13	0.4	385	1	1 Starch, 2 Lean Meat, 2 1/2 Fat
Batter-dipped, drumstick	1 whole	193	11	3	6	0.2	194	1/2	1/2 Starch, 2 Lean Meat, 1 Fat
Batter-dipped, thigh	1 whole	238	14	3.8	8	0.3	248	1/2	3/4 Starch, 2 Lean Meat, 2 1/2 Fat
Batter-dipped, wing	1 whole	159	11	2.9	5	0.1	157	0	1/2 Starch, 1 Lean Meat, 2 Fat
Flour-coated, breast	1/2 breast	218	9	2.4	2	0.1	74	0	1/2 Starch, 4 Lean Meat, 1 Fat
Flour-coated, drumstick	1 whole	120	7	1.8	1	Tr	44	0	1-1/2 Lean Meat, 1/2 Fat
Meat only, dark meat	1 oz	68	3.3	1	1	0	27	0	1 Medium-Fat Meat
Meat only, light meat	1 oz	54	2	0.5	Tr	0	23	0	1 Medium-Fat Meat

	Portion	Cal	Fat (g)	Sat Fat (g)	Carb (g)	Fiber (g)	Sod (mgs)	Carb Choices	Exchanges
Roasted, breast, meat only	1/2 breast	142	3	0.9	0	0	64	0	2 Lean Meat
Roasted, drumstick, meat only	1 whole	76	2	0.7	0	0	42	0	1 Medium-Fat Meat
Roasted, thigh, meat only	1 whole	109	6	1.6	0	0	46	0	1 1/2 Medium-Fat Meat
Stewed, meat only, light and dark	1 cup	332	17	4.3	0	0	109	0	6 1/2 Very Lean Meat, 2 1/2 Fat
Chicken, giblets, simmered	1 cup	228	7	2.2	1	0	84	0	6 Very Lean Meat, 3/4 Fat
Chicken, liver, simmered	1 piece	31	1	0.4	Tr	0	10	0	3/4 Lean Meat, 1/4 Fat
Chicken neck, meat only	1 neck	32	1	0.4	0	0	12	0	1 Lean Meat
Duck									
Roasted, flesh only	1/2 duck	444	25	9.2	0	0	144	0	8 Lean Meat
Turkey									
Roasted, meat only, dark	1 oz	53	2	1	0	0	22	0	1 Lean Meat
Roasted, meat only, light	1 oz	44	1	0.3	0	0	18	0	1 Very Lean Meat
Roasted, light and dark, chopped	1 cup	238	7	2.3	0	0	98	0	6 Very Lean Meat, 3/4 Fat
Ground, cooked, from 4oz raw	1 patty	193	11	2.8	0	0	88	0	3 Lean Meat, 1/3 Fat

	Portion	Cal	Fat (g)	Sat Fat (g)	Carb (g)	Fiber (g)	Sod (mgs)	Carb Choices	Exchanges
Ground, cooked, crumbled	1 cup	298	17	4.3	0	0	136	0	5 Lean Meat, 1/2 Fat
Turkey giblets, simmered	1 cup	242	7	2.2	3	0	86	0	6 Very Lean Meat, 3/4 Fat
Turkey neck, meat only, simmered	1 neck	274	11	3.7	0	0	85	0	5 Lean Meat
Poultry Food Products									
Chicken, canned, boneless	1 oz	47	2	1	0	0	143	0	1 Lean Meat
Chicken frankfurter	1 frank	116	9	2.5	3	0	617	0	1 High-Fat Meat
Chicken roll, light meat	1 slice	45	2	0.5	0.5	0	166	0	1 High-Fat Meat
Turkey and gravy, frozen	5 oz pkg	95	4	1.2	7	0	787	1/2	1/2 Starch, 1 Lean Meat
Turkey patties, breaded, fried	1 patty	181	12	3	10	0.3	512	1/2	1/2 Starch, 1 Lean Meat, 1 1/2 Fat
Turkey roast, boneless, frozen	1 oz	44	2	0.5	1	0	193	0	1 Very Lean Meat, 1/4 Fat
Beef, cooked									
Braised, simmered, or pot-roasted									
Chuck blade, lean and fat	1 oz	98	7	2.9	0	0	18	0	1 High-Fat Meat

	Portion	Cal	Fat (g)	Sat Fat (g)	Carb (g)	Fiber (g)	Sod (mgs)	Carb Choices	Exchanges
Chuck blade, lean only	1 oz	71	4	1.4	0	0	20	0	1 Medium-Fat Meat
Bottom round, lean and fat	1 oz	78	5	1.8	0	0	14	0	1 Medium-Fat Meat
Bottom round, lean only	1 oz	59	2	0.8	0	0	14	0	1 Lean Meat
Ground beef, broiled									
83% lean	1 oz	73	5	1.8	0	0	20	0	1 Medium-Fat Meat
79% lean	1 oz	77	5	2	0	0	22	0	1 Medium-Fat Meat
73% lean	1 oz	82	6	2.3	0	0	24	0	1 High-Fat Meat
Liver, fried, sliced	1 oz	61	2	0.8	7	0	30	0.5	1 Lean Meat
Roast, oven-cooked, no liquid									
Rib, lean and fat	1 oz	101	8	3.3	0	0	18	0	1 High-Fat Meat
Rib, lean only	1 oz	65	4	1.4	0	0	20	0	1 Medium-Fat Meat
Eye round, lean and fat	1 oz	65	4	1.4	0	0	17	0	1 Medium-Fat Meat
Eye round, lean only	1 oz	48	1	0.5	0	0	18	0	1 Very Lean Meat
Steak, sirloin, broiled, lean and fat	1 oz	73	4	1.7	0	0	18	0	1 Medium-Fat Meat

	Portion	Cal	Fat (g)	Sat Fat (g)	Carb (g)	Fiber (g)	Sod (mgs)	Carb Choices	Exchanges
Steak, sirloin, broiled, lean only	1 oz	55	2	0.8	0	0	19	0	1 Lean Meat
Beef, canned, corned	1 oz	71	4	1.7	0	0	285	0	1 Medium-Fat Meat
Beef, dried, chipped	1 oz	16	Tr	Tr	Tr	0	328	0	1/2 Very Lean Meat
Lamb, cooked									
Chops, arm, braised, lean and fat	1 oz	98	7	2.8	0	0	20	0	1 High-Fat Meat
Chops, arm, braised, lean only	1 oz	79	4	1.4	0	0	22	0	1 Medium-Fat Meat
Lamb, cooked									
Chops, loin, broiled, lean and fat	1 oz	90	7	2.8	0	0	22	0	1 High-Fat Meat
Chops, loin, broiled, lean only	1 oz	61	3	1	0	0	24	0	1 Lean Meat
Leg, roasted, lean and fat	1 oz	73	5	2	0	0	19	0	1 Medium-Fat Meat
Leg, roasted, lean only	1 oz	54	2	0.7	0	0	19	0	1 Lean Meat
Rib, roasted, lean and fat	1 oz	102	8	3.6	0	0	21	0	1 High-Fat Meat
Rib, roasted, lean only	1 oz	66	4	1.3	0	0	23	0	1 Medium-Fat Meat

	Portion	Cal	Fat (g)	Sat Fat (g)	Carb (g)	Fiber (g)	Sod (mgs)	Carb Choices	Exchanges
Pork, cured, cooked									
Bacon, regular	3 slices	109	9	3.3	Tr	0	303	0	1High-Fat Meat
Bacon, streaky, raw	1 oz	154	16	5.9	0	0	190	0	1 High-Fat Meat, 1 Fat
Bacon, streaky, cooked	1 oz	160	13.6	4.8	0	0	443	0	1 High-Fat Meat, 1 Fat
Bacon, Canadian-style	1 oz	43	2	0.7	Tr	0	240	0	1 Lean Meat
Ham, roasted, lean and fat	1 oz	69	5	1.7	0	0	336	0	1 Medium-Fat Meat
Ham, roasted, lean only	1 oz	44	2	0.5	0	0	376	0	1 Lean Meat
Ham, canned, roasted	1 oz	47	2	0.8	Tr	0	303	0	1 Lean Meat
Pork, fresh, cooked									
Chop, loin, broiled, lean and fat	1 oz	68	4	1.4	0	0	16	0	1 Medium-Fat Meat
Chop, loin, broiled, lean only	1 oz	57	2	0.8	0	0	17	0	1 Lean Meat
Chop, loin, pan-fried, lean and fat	1 oz	78	5	1.7	0	0	23	0	1 Medium-Fat Meat
Chop, loin, pan-fried, lean only	1 oz	66	3	1	0	0	24	0	1 Lean Meat

	Portion	Cal	Fat (g)	Sat Fat (g)	Carb (g)	Fiber (g)	Sod (mgs)	Carb Choices	Exchanges
Ham, leg, roasted, lean and fat	1 oz	77	5	1.8	0	0	17	0	1 Medium-Fat Meat
Ham, leg, roasted, lean only	1 oz	60	3	1	0	0	18	0	1 Lean Meat
Rib roast, lean and fat	1 oz	72	4	1.6	0	0	13	0	1 Medium-Fat Meat
Rib roast, lean only	1 oz	63	3	1.2	0	0	13	0	1 Lean Meat
Pork, fresh, cooked									
Ribs, back ribs, roasted	1 oz	105	8	3.1	0	0	29	0	1 High-Fat Meat
Ribs, country-style, braised	1 oz	84	6	2.3	0	0	17	0	1 Medium-Fat Meat
Ribs, spareribs, braised	1 oz	112	9	3.2	0	0	26	0	1 High-Fat Meat
Shoulder cut, braised, lean and fat	1 oz	93	7	2.4	0	0	25	0	1 High-Fat Meat
Shoulder cut, braised, lean only	1 oz	70	3	1.2	0	0	29	0	1 Medium-Fat Meat
Sausages and Luncheon Meats									
Bologna, beef and pork	1 slice	90	8	3	2	0	290	0	1 High-Fat Meat
Braunschweiger	1 slice	103	9	3.1	2	0	326	0	1 High-Fat Meat

	Portion	Cal	Fat (g)	Sat Fat (g)	Carb (g)	Fiber (g)	Sod (mgs)	Carb Choices	Exchanges
Brown and serve, cooked	2 links	103	9	3.4	1	0	209	0	1 High-Fat Meat
Canned, minced luncheon meat	1 slice	86	8	2.5	1	0	270	0	1 High-Fat Meat
Chopped ham	1 oz	32	3	0.8	0	0	192	0	1 Lean Meat
Cooked ham, regular	1 slice	52	3	1	1	0	376	0	1 Lean Meat
Cooked ham, extra lean	1 slice	38	1.5	0.5	0.5	0	408	0	1 Very Lean Meat
Frankfurter, beef and pork	1 frank	144	13	4.8	1	0	504	0	1 1/2 High-Fat Meat
Frankfurter, beef	1 frank	142	13	5.4	1	0	462	0	1 1/2 High-Fat Meat
Pork sausage, fresh, cooked, links	2 links	96	8	2.8	Tr	0	336	0	1 High-Fat Meat
Pork sausage, fresh, cooked, patty	1 patty	100	8	2.9	Tr	0	349	0	1 High-Fat Meat
Salami, beef and pork, cooked type	1 slice	72	5.5	2.3	0.5	0	304	0	1 Medium-Fat Meat
Salami, beef and pork, dry type	1 slice	42	3.5	1.2	0.5	0	186	0	1 Lean Meat
Sandwich spread, pork, beef	1 Tbsp	35	3	0.9	2	Tr	152	0	1 Very Lean Meat
Vienna sausage	1 sausage	45	4	1.5	Tr	0	152	0	1 Lean Meat

	Portion	Cal	Fat (g)	Sat Fat (g)	Carb (g)	Fiber (g)	Sod (mgs)	Carb Choices	Exchanges
Veal, lean and fat, cooked									
Cutlet, braised	1 oz	60	2	0.7	0	0	19	0	1 Lean Meat
Rib, roasted	1 oz	65	4	1.5	0	0	26	0	1 Medium-Fat Meat
Offals									
Brain, beef, raw	1 oz	35	2.6	0.6	0	0	29	0	1 Lean Meat
Feet, trotters									
Pork, medium fat	1 oz	79	6	0	0	0	0	0	1 Medium-Fat Meat
Heart									
Beef	1 oz	33	1	0.3	0.7	0	18	0	1 Very Lean Meat
Mutton or lamb	1 oz	34	1.6	0.6	0	0	25	0	1 Very Lean Meat
Pork	1 oz	33	1.2	0.3	0.4	0	16	0	1 Very Lean Meat
Intestine or tripe									
Beef	1 oz	27	1.1	0.5	0	0	13	0	1 Very Lean Meat
Pork	1 oz	44	2.6	0	0	0	14	0	1 Lean Meat
Kidney									
Beef	1 oz	30	1	0.3	0.6	0	50	0	1 Very Lean Meat
Mutton or lamb	1 oz	27	1	0.3	0.2	0	43	0	1 Very Lean Meat
Pork	1 oz	28	1	0.3	0	0	34	0	1 Very Lean Meat

	Portion	Cal	Fat (g)	Sat Fat (g)	Carb (g)	Fiber (g)	Sod (mgs)	Carb Choices	Exchanges
Liver									
Beef, raw	1 oz	40	1	0.4	1.6	0	20	0	1 Very Lean Meat
Beef, stewed	1 oz	45	1.4	0.5	1	0	19	0	1 Very Lean Meat
Chicken, raw	1 oz	38	1.8	0.5	0.2	0	24	0	1 Very Lean Meat
Mutton or lamb, raw	1 oz	39	1.4	0.5	0.5	0	19	0	1 Very Lean Meat
Pork, raw	1 oz	37	1	0.3	0.7	0	24	0	1 Very Lean Meat
Pork, cooked	1 oz	46	1.2	0.4	1	0	14	0	1 Very Lean Meat
Lung									
Beef	1 oz	26	0.7	0.3	0	0	55	0	1 Very Lean Meat
Mutton or lamb	1 oz	26	0.7	0	0	0	44	0	1 Very Lean Meat
Pork	1 oz	24	0.8	0.3	0	0	43	0	1 Very Lean Meat
Tail									
Ox, lean only, raw	1 oz	48	2.8	0	0	0	31	0	1 Lean Meat
Stewed (salt added)	1 oz	68	3.7	0	0	0	53	0	1 Lean Meat
Pig, in brine	1 oz	119	11.6	0	0	0	0	0	1 High-Fat Meat, 1/2 Fat
Pig, fresh	1 oz	105	9.3	3.2	0	0	0	0	1 High-Fat Meat
Pork trotters and tails, salted/boiled	1 oz	78	6.2	0	0	0	449	0	1 Medium-Fat Meat

	Portion	Cal	Fat (g)	Sat Fat (g)	Carb (g)	Fiber (g)	Sod (mgs)	Carb Choices	Exchanges
Tongue									
Beef, fresh, raw	1 oz	62	4.5	1.9	1	0	19	0	1 Medium-Fat Meat
Pickled, boiled (fat and skin removed)	1 oz	81	6.6	0	0	0	278	0	1 Medium-Fat Meat
Mutton or lamb, fresh, raw	1 oz	62	4.8	1.8	0	0	22	0	1 Medium-Fat Meat
Pork, fresh, raw	1 oz	63	4.8	1.6	0	0	31	0	1 Medium-Fat Meat
Black pudding, fried	1 oz	85	6	2.4	0	0	336	0	1 Medium-Fat Meat
Other Meats and Game									
Goat, raw	1 oz	30	0.6	0	0	0	0	0	1 Very Lean Meat
Mammals, dressed	1 oz	34	1	0	0	0	0	0	1 Very Lean Meat
Birds, dressed	1 oz	40	1.4	0	0	0	0	0	1 Very Lean Meat
Guinea pig, flesh only	1 oz	27	0.4	0	0	0	0	0	1 Very Lean Meat
Iguana	1 oz	31	0	0	0	0	0	0	1 Very Lean Meat
Rabbit, flesh, raw	1 oz	38	1.5	0.5	0	0	11	0	1 Very Lean Meat
Rabbit, flesh, stewed	1 oz	50	2.1	0	0	0	9	0	1 Very Lean Meat
Cheeses, Natural									
Blue cheese	1 oz	100	8	5.3	1	0	396	0	1 High-Fat Meat

	Portion	Cal	Fat (g)	Sat Fat (g)	Carb (g)	Fiber (g)	Sod (mgs)	Carb Choices	Exchanges
Camembert	1 oz	85	7	4.3	Tr	0	239	0	1 High-Fat Meat
Cheddar, cut pieces	1 oz	114	9	6	Tr	0	173	0	1 High-Fat Meat
Cheddar, shredded	1 cup	455	37	23.8	1	0	701	0	4 High-Fat Meat
Cheddar or colby, low-fat	1 oz	49	2	1.2	1	0	174	0	1 Lean Meat
Cottage Cheeses									
Creamed, 4% fat, large curd	1 cup	233	10	6.4	6	0	911	1/2	4 Lean Meat
Creamed, 4% fat, small curd	1 cup	217	9	6	6	0	850	1/2	4 Lean Meat
Creamed, 4% fat, w/ fruit	1 cup	279	8	4.9	30	0	915	2	3 Lean Meat, 2 Starch
Creamed, low-fat (2%)	1 cup	203	4	2.8	8	0	918	1/2	4 Very Lean Meat
Creamed, low-fat (1%)	1 cup	164	2	1.5	6	0	918	1/2	4 Very Lean Meat
Uncreamed, less than 1/2% fat	1 cup	123	1	0.4	3	0	19	0	4 Very Lean Meat
Feta	1 oz	75	6	4.2	1	0	316	0	1 Medium-Fat Meat
Mozzarella, part skim milk	1 oz	79	5	3.1	1	0	150	0	1 Medium-Fat Meat
Mozzarella, whole milk	1 oz	80	6	3.7	1	0	106	0	1 Medium-Fat Meat

	Portion	Cal	Fat (g)	Sat Fat (g)	Carb (g)	Fiber (g)	Sod (mgs)	Carb Choices	Exchanges
Muenster	1 oz	104	9	5.4	Tr	0	178	0	1 High-Fat Meat
Parmesan, grated	1 cup	456	30	19.1	4	0	1,862	0	8 Lean Meat
Parmesan, grated	1 Tbsp	23	2	1	Tr	0	93	0	1/2 Lean Meat
Parmesan, grated	1 oz	129	9	5.4	1	0	528	0	4 Lean Meat
Provolone	1 oz	100	8	4.8	1	0	248	0	1 High-Fat Meat
Ricotta, part skim milk	1 cup	340	19	12.1	13	0	307	1/2	4 High-Fat Meat
Ricotta, whole milk	1 cup	428	32	20.4	7	0	207	1	4 Medium-Fat Meat
Swiss, natural	1 oz	107	8	5	1	0	74	0	1 High-Fat Meat
Cheeses, Pasteurized Processed									
American, fat-free	1 slice	31	Tr	0.1	3	0	321	0	1 Very Lean Meat
American, regular	1 oz	106	9	5.6	Tr	0	406	0	1 High-Fat Meat
American, cheese food	1 oz	93	7	4.4	2	0	337	0	1 High-Fat Meat
American, spread	1 oz	82	6	3.8	2	0	381	0	1 High-Fat Meat
Swiss	1 oz	95	7	4.5	1	0	388	0	1 High-Fat Meat
Eggs									
Whole, raw	1 medium	66	4	1.4	1	0	55	0	1 Medium-Fat Meat

	Portion	Cal	Fat (g)	Sat Fat (g)	Carb (g)	Fiber (g)	Sod (mgs)	Carb Choices	Exchanges
Whole, raw	1 large	75	5	1.6	1	0	63	0	1 Medium-Fat Meat
Whole, raw	1 extra large	86	6	1.8	1	0	73	0	1 Medium-Fat Meat
White, raw	1 large	17	0	0	Tr	0	55	0	1/2 Very Lean Meat
Yolk, raw	1 large	59	5	1.6	Tr	0	7	0	1 Medium-Fat Meat
Whole, fried, margarine and salt	1 large	92	7	1.9	1	0	162	0	1 Medium-Fat Meat, 1/2 Fat
Hard-cooked, shell removed	1 large	78	5	1.6	1	0	62	0	1 Medium-Fat Meat
Hard-cooked, chopped	1 cup	211	14	4.4	2	0	169	0	3 Medium-Fat Meat
Poached, with salt	1 large	75	5	1.5	1	0	140	0	1 Medium-Fat Meat
Scrambled, margarine, salt, milk	1 large	101	7	2.2	1	0	171	0	1 Medium-Fat Meat, 1/2 Fat
Egg substitute, liquid	1/4 cup	53	2	0.4	Tr	0	112	0	1 Very Lean Meat

Chapter 20

Fats Choices

Oils, nuts, and solid fats are part of the fat group. Foods that are mainly oil include mayonnaise, certain salad dressings, and soft (tub or squeeze) margarine with no trans fats. Most oils are high in monounsaturated or polyunsaturated fats and low in saturated fats. However, coconut oil and palm kernel oil are high in saturated fats. Oils from plant sources like vegetable and nut oils do not contain any cholesterol.

Dietary Guidelines suggest you limit your fat intake to less than 10% of calories from saturated fat and less than 300 mg of cholesterol daily, and keep trans fats as low as possible.

Fats Tips:

- ⦿ Make most of your fat sources from fish, nuts, and vegetable oils.

- ⦿ Limit solid fats like butter, stick margarine, shortening, and lard, as well as foods that contain these.

- ⦿ Check the Nutrition Facts Label to keep saturated fats and trans fats low.

FATS CHOICES

	Portion	Cal	Fat (g)	Sat Fat (g)	Carb (g)	Fiber (g)	Sod (mgs)	Carb Choices	Exchanges
MONOUNSATURATED									
Almonds, whole	8 nuts	55	5	0.4	2	1.1	Tr	0	1 Fat
Avocados, California, raw	1 oz	50	5	0.7	2	1.4	3	0	1 Fat
Avocados, Florida, raw	1 oz	32	3	0.5	3	1.5	1	0	1/2 Fat
Cashews, salted, dry roasted	7 nuts	63	5	1	3.4	0.4	70	0	1 Fat
Cashews, salted, oil roasted	7 nuts	58	5	1	2.8	0.4	63	0	1 Fat
Creamer, sweet, liquid, frozen	1 Tbsp	20	1	0.3	2	0	12	0	0 Fat
Lard	1 Tbsp	115	13	5	0	0	Tr	0	2 1/2 Fat
Macadamia nuts	3 nuts	46	5	0.8	0.9	0.5	17	0	1 Fat
Margarine, hard	1 Tbsp	101	11	2.2	Tr	0	132	0	2 Fat
Margarine, spread	1 Tbsp	51	6	1.2	Tr	0	138	0	1 Fat
Margarine, butter blend	1 Tbsp	102	11	4	Tr	0	127	0	2 Fat
Peanuts, dry roasted, salted	10 nuts	59	5	0.7	2	0.8	82	0	1 Fat
Peanuts, dry roasted, unsalted	10 nuts	59	5	0.7	2	0.8	Tr	0	1 Fat
Peanuts, oil roasted, salted	10 nuts	59	5	0.7	1.8	0.9	44	0	1 Fat
Peanut butter, regular, smooth	2 tsp	59	5	1	1.9	0.6	47	0	1 Fat
Peanut butter, regular, chunky	2 tsp	59	5	1	1.9	0.7	49	0	1 Fat
Peanut butter, reduced-fat	2 1/2 tsp	78	5	1	5	0.8	81	0	1 Fat

	Portion	Cal	Fat (g)	Sat Fat (g)	Carb (g)	Fiber (g)	Sod (mgs)	Carb Choices	Exchanges
Pecans	5 halves	49	5	0.5	4	2.6	0	0	1 Fat
Pine nuts	1 Tbsp	49	4	0.7	1	0.4	Tr	0	1 Fat
Pistachio nuts	18 nuts	62	5	0.6	3	1	47	0	1 Fat
Oils									
Canola	1 Tbsp	124	14	1	0	0	0	0	3 Fat
Olive	1 Tbsp	119	14	1.8	0	0	Tr	0	3 Fat
Peanut	1 Tbsp	119	14	2.3	0	0	Tr	0	3 Fat
Safflower	1 Tbsp	120	14	0.8	0	0	0	0	3 Fat
Soybean, hydrogenated	1 Tbsp	120	14	2	0	0	0	0	3 Fat
Salad dressing, homemade									
Made w/margarine	1 Tbsp	25	2	0.5	2	0	117	0	1/2 Fat
W/Shortening	1 Tbsp	113	13	3.2	0	0	0	0	3 Fat
POLYUNSATURATED									
Brazil nuts	2 nuts	49	2	1.2	1	0.4	0	0	1 Fat
Mayonnaise									
Regular	1 Tbsp	99	11	1.6	Tr	0	78	0	2 Fat
Light, cholesterol-free	1 Tbsp	49	5	0.7	1	0	107	0	1 Fat
Fat-free	1 Tbsp	12	Tr	0.1	2	0.6	190	0	0 Fat
Margarine, soft	1 Tbsp	102	12	2	Tr	0	153	0	2 1/2 Fat
Oils									
Corn	1 Tbsp	120	14	1.7	0	0	0	0	3 Fat
Sesame	1 Tbsp	120	14	1.9	0	0	0	0	3 Fat
Soybean/cottonseed blend	1 Tbsp	120	14	2.4	0	0	0	0	3 Fat
Sunflower	1 Tbsp	120	14	1.4	0	0	0	0	3 Fat
Pumpkin and squash seeds	60 seeds	62	5	1	1.7	0.5	68	0	1 Fat

	Portion	Cal	Fat (g)	Sat Fat (g)	Carb (g)	Fiber (g)	Sod (mgs)	Carb Choices	Exchanges
Salad dressing, commercial									
Bleu cheese, regular	1 Tbsp	77	8	1.5	1	0	167	0	1 Fat
Bleu cheese, lo-cal	1 Tbsp	15	1	0.4	Tr	0	184	0	0 Fat
Caesar, regular	1 Tbsp	78	8	1.3	Tr	Tr	158	0	1 Fat
Caesar, lo-cal	1 Tbsp	17	1	0.1	3	Tr	162	0	0 Fat
French, regular	1 Tbsp	67	6	1.5	3	0	214	0	1 Fat
French, lo-cal	1 Tbsp	22	1	0.1	4	0	128	0	0 Fat
Italian, regular	1 Tbsp	69	7	1	1	0	116	0	1 Fat
Italian, lo-cal	1 Tbsp	16	1	0.2	1	Tr	118	0	0 Fat
Russian, regular	1 Tbsp	76	8	1.1	2	0	133	0	1 Fat
Russian, lo-cal	1 Tbsp	23	1	0.1	4	Tr	141	0	0 Fat
Thousand island, regular	1 Tbsp	59	6	0.9	2	0	109	0	1 Fat
Thousand island, lo-cal	1 Tbsp	24	2	0.2	2	0.2	153	0	0 Fat
Salad dressing, homemade									
French	1 Tbsp	88	10	1.8	Tr	0	92	0	2 Fat
Vinegar and oil	1 Tbsp	70	8	1.4	Tr	0	Tr	0	1 Fat
Sunflower seeds	1 Tbsp	58	5	0.5	2.5	0.9	78	0	1 Fat
Tahini	1 Tbsp	89	8	1.1	3	1.4	17	0	1 1/2 Fat
Walnuts	4 halves	51	5	0.5	1	0.5	0	0	1 Fat
SATURATED									
Butter, salted	1 Tbsp	102	12	7.2	Tr	0	117	0	3 Fat
Butter, unsalted	1 Tbsp	102	12	7.2	Tr	0	1.5	0	3 Fat
Cream cheese, regular	1 oz	99	10	6.2	1	0	84	0	2 Fat
Cream cheese, regular	1 Tbsp	51	5	3.2	Tr	0	43	0	1 Fat
Cream cheese, low-fat	1 Tbsp	35	3	1.7	1	0	44	0	1/2 Fat
Cream cheese, fat-free	1 Tbsp	15	Tr	0.1	1	0	85	0	0 Fat

	Portion	Cal	Fat (g)	Sat Fat (g)	Carb (g)	Fiber (g)	Sod (mgs)	Carb Choices	Exchanges
Cream, sweet									
Half-and-half	1 Tbsp	20	2	1.1	1	0	6	0	1/2 Fat
Light	1 Tbsp	29	3	1.8	1	0	6	0	1/2 Fat
Whipping (unwhipped)									
Light	1 Tbsp	44	5	2.9	Tr	0	5	0	1 Fat
Heavy	1 Tbsp	52	6	3.5	Tr	0	6	0	1 Fat
Whipped topping, pressurized	1 Tbsp	8	1	0.4	Tr	0	4	0	0 Fat
Cream, sour									
Regular	1 Tbsp	26	3	1.6	1	0	6	0	1/2 Fat
Reduced-fat	1 Tbsp	20	2	1.1	1	0	6	0	1/2 Fat
Fat-free	1 Tbsp	12	0	0	2	0	23	0	0 Fat
Creamer, sweet, powdered	1 tsp	11	1	0.7	1	0	4	0	0 Fat
Ghee, butter	1 tsp	42	4.7	3	0	0	0.1	0	1 Fat
Lard/leaf fat	1 tsp	39	4.3	1.8	Tr	0	0.1	0	1 Fat
Meat fat									
Beef	1 tsp	39	4.3	2	0	0	0	0	1 Fat
Mutton, tallow	1 tsp	39	4.3	2	0	0	0	0	1 Fat
Pork	1 tsp	39	4.3	1.7	0	0	0	0	1 Fat
Neufchatel	1 oz	74	7	4.2	1	0	113	0	1 Fat, 1/2 Lean Meat
Oil, coconut	1 tsp	42	4.7	0.84	0	0	Tr	0	1 Fat
Oil, cottonseed	1 tsp	42	4.7	0.84	0	0	Tr	0	1 Fat
Palm oil, red	1 tsp	41	4.7	2.3	0	0	0	0	1 Fat
Palm oil, kernel	1 tsp	41	4.7	3.8	0	0	0	0	1 Fat
Sour dressing	1 Tbsp	21	2	1.6	1	0	6	0	1/2 Fat
Whipped topping									
Frozen	1 Tbsp	13	1	0.9	1	0	1	0	0 Fat

	Portion	Cal	Fat (g)	Sat Fat (g)	Carb (g)	Fiber (g)	Sod (mgs)	Carb Choices	Exchanges
Powder, prepared w/ whole milk	1 Tbsp	8	Tr	0.4	1	0	3	0	0 Fat

Chapter 21

Free Food Choices

Spices and condiments are part of the free food list. These foods do not add significant amounts of carbohydrates or calories to the diet.

Spice and Condiment Tip:

🍽 Pay attention to the sodium content.

FREE FOOD CHOICES

	Portion	Cal	Fat (g)	Sat Fat (g)	Carb (g)	Fiber (g)	Sod (mgs)	Carb Choices	Exchanges
Spices and Condiments									
Barbecue sauce	1 Tbsp	13	0.3	0	2.2	0.1	138	0	Free Food
Cinnamon bark, ground	1 tsp	5	0	0	1.8	0.5	0	0	Free Food
Chili powder	1 tsp	8	0.4	0	1.4	0.6	25	0	Free Food
Coriander seed	1 tsp	5	0.3	0	0.9	0.5	1	0	Free Food
Curry powder	1 tsp	8	0.3	0	1.5	0.4	1.3	0	Free Food
Fennel seed	1 tsp	7	0.3	0	1	0.3	1.7	0	Free Food
Garlic, fresh bulb, raw	1 clove	4	0	0	1	0	0.5	0	Free Food
Ginger									
Root, fresh	1 slice	2	0	0	0.3	0	0.3	0	Free Food
Root, dried, ground	1 tsp	9	0.2	0	1.8	0	1	0	Free Food
Fish sauce	1 Tbsp								Free Food
Hot pepper sauce	1 Tbsp	3	0	0	0	0.7	0.1	0	Free Food
Ketchup	1 Tbsp	5	0	0	1.2	0.1	103	0	Free Food
Mint	1 tsp	0	0	0	0	0	0	0	Free Food
Mustard, prepared, yellow	1 Tbsp	13	0.8	0	1	0.2	212	0	Free Food
Parsley	1 tsp	0	0	0	0	0	0	0	Free Food

	Portion	Cal	Fat (g)	Sat Fat (g)	Carb (g)	Fiber (g)	Sod (mgs)	Carb Choices	Exchanges
Pepper, dry, black	1 tsp	5	0	0	0	1.3	0.3	1	Free Food
Pimento leaf	1 tsp								Free Food
Salt, table	1 tsp	0	0	0	0	0	2334	0	Free Food
Soya sauce	1 Tbsp	10	0	0	0	1.2	866	0	Free Food
Thyme leaf, ground	1 tsp	1	0	0	0	0.2	0	0	Free Food
Tomato chili sauce, bottled	1 Tbsp	6	0	0	1.2	0	80	0	Free Food
Turmeric	1 tsp	8	0.2	0	0	1.5	1	0	Free Food
Vinegar	1 Tbsp	2	0	0	0	0.8	0	0	Free Food

Chapter 22

Sweets and Dessert Choices

Sweets and desserts can be included in a healthy diet. Some sweets, like cakes, pies, and cookies, are also high in saturated fat and trans fat. Most of the calories in these foods come from carbohydrates and fat. Talk to your registered dietitian (RD) or certified diabetes educator (CDE) about how to fit sweet foods into your meal plan.

Sweets and dessert tips:

- Keep the amount of sweets and desserts within your carbohydrate allowance by substituting sweets and desserts for starch fruit or milk choices.

- Choose low-fat or fat-free desserts with caution; they often have more total carbohydrates.

- Control portion sizes.

- Limit sweets and dessert choices to one per day.

SWEETS AND DESSERT CHOICES

	Portion	Cal	Fat (g)	Sat Fat (g)	Carb (g)	Fiber (g)	Sod (mgs)	Carb Choices	Exchanges
Angel food cake, unfrosted	1/12 cake	72	0	0	16	0.4	210	1	1 CHO
Brownie, unfrosted	2 3/4" sq	227	9	2.4	36	1.2	175	2 1/2	2 CHO, 2 Fat
Brownie, fat-free	2" sq	89	Tr	0.2	22	1	90	1 1/2	1 CHO
Cake, chocolate, unfrosted	1/12 of 9"	340	14	5	51	1.5	299	3 1/2	3 CHO, 1 Fat
Cake, yellow w/choc frosting	1/12 of 9"	243	9	1.5	35	1.2	216	2	2 CHO, 2 Fat
Candy									
Caramel, plain	1 piece	39	1	0.7	8	0.1	25	1/2	1/2 CHO
Carob	1 oz	153	9	8.2	16	1.1	30	1	1 CHO, 1 Fat
Chocolate bar									
Plain, milk	1 each	226	14	8.1	26	1.5	36	2	2 CHO, 2 Fat
With almonds	1 each	216	14	7	22	2.5	30	1 1/2	1 1/2 CHO, 2 1/2 Fat
Chocolate chips									
Milk	1 cup	862	52	31	99	5.7	138	7	7 CHO, 7 Fat
Semisweet	1 cup	805	50	30	106	9.9	18	8	7 CHO, 7 Fat
White	1 cup	916	55	33	101	0	153	7 1/2	7 CHO, 8 Fat

	Portion	Cal	Fat (g)	Sat Fat (g)	Carb (g)	Fiber (g)	Sod (mgs)	Carb Choices	Exchanges
Chocolate-coated peanuts	10 pcs	208	13	6	20	1.9	16	1	1 CHO, 2 1/2 Fat
Chocolate-coated raisins	10 pcs	39	1	1	7	0.4	4	1/2	1/2 CHO
Fruit leather	1 sm. roll	49	Tr	0.1	12	0.5	9	1	1 CHO
Fudge, plain	1 piece	65	1	1	14	0.1	11	1	1 CHO
Fudge, with nuts	1 piece	81	3	1.1	14	0.2	11	1	1 CHO, 1/2 Fat
Gum drops	1 cup	703	0	0	180	0	80	12	12 CHO
Hard candy	1 piece	24	0	0	6	0	2	1/2	1/2 CHO
Jelly beans	10 small	40	0	0	10	0	3	1/2	1/2 CHO
Cookies									
Butter	1 cookie	23	1	0.6	3	Tr	18	0	1/4 CHO
Chocolate Chip	1 cookie	48	2	0.7	7	0.3	32	1/2	1/2 CHO, 1/2 Fat
Oatmeal	1 cookie	61	2	0.5	10	0.4	52	1/2	1/2 CHO, 1/2 Fat
Sandwich type, cream-filled	1 cookie	47	2	0.4	7	0.3	60	1/2	1/2 CHO, 1/2 Fat
Shortbread, plain	1 cookie	40	2	0.5	5	0.1	36	0	1/2 CHO, 1/2 Fat
Sugar	1 cookie	72	3	0.8	10	0.1	54	1/2	1/2 CHO, 1/2 Fat
Custard	1/2 cup	148	4	2	23	0	118	1 1/2	1 1/2 CHO, 1 Fat
Danish, cheese-filled	1 each	266	16	4.8	26	0.7	320	2	2 CHO, 3 Fat
Danish, fruit-filled	1 each	263	13	3.5	34	1.3	251	2	2 1/2 CHO, 2 Fat

	Portion	Cal	Fat (g)	Sat Fat (g)	Carb (g)	Fiber (g)	Sod (mgs)	Carb Choices	Exchanges
Doughnut, glazed	1 medium	242	14	3.5	27	0.7	205	2	2 CHO, 3 Fat
Doughnut, plain cake	1 medium	198	11	1.7	23	0.7	257	1 1/2	1 1/2 CHO, 2 Fat
Fruit juice bars, 100% juice	1 bar	63	0	0	16	0	3	1	1 CHO
Gelatin, regular	1/2 cup	80	0	0	19	0	57	1	1 CHO
Granola bar	1 bar	134	6	0.7	18	1.5	83	1	1 CHO, 1 Fat
Honey	1 Tbsp	64	0	0	17	0	1	1	1 CHO
Jam or Jelly	1 Tbsp	55	0	0	14	0.2	6	1	1 CHO
Marshmallows	1 regular	23	Tr	Tr	6	Tr	3	1/2	1/2 CHO
Pie, fruit, 2 crusts	1/6 pie	277	13	4.4	40	1.9	311	2 1/2	3 CHO, 2 Fat
Pie, pumpkin or custard	1/8 pie	316	14	4.9	41	2.9	349	3	2 CHO, 2 Fat
Pudding, prepared with 2% milk	1/2 cup	150	3	1.6	28	0.6	417	2	2 CHO
Soft drink/ Soda pop	6 oz	76	0	0	19	0	7	1	1 1/2 CHO
Sports drink	8 oz	225	0	0	15	0	96	1	1 CHO
Sugar	1 Tbsp	48	0	0	18	0	0	1	1 CHO
Syrup, light	1 Tbsp	25	0	0	7	0	30	1/2	1/2 CHO
Syrup, regular	1 Tbsp	57	0	0	15	0	17	1	1 CHO

Chapter 23

Combination Food and Fast Food Choices

Combination food and fast foods often fit into more than one food group. Caution should be used when choosing mixed dishes and particularly fast foods: they are generally high in calories, sodium, and fat.

Most fast food restaurants offer healthy options and will provide you with the nutrient information for foods on their menu.

Fast Food Tips:

- Have it your way and ask for burgers and sandwiches without added sauces or toppings.

- Substitute a side salad for French fries.

- Choose grilled or flame-broiled sandwiches and burgers.

- Don't super-size your order.

- Choose the kids meal.

- Have fruit for dessert.

- Choose low-fat milk, water, or diet soda for your beverage.

COMBINATION FOOD and FAST FOOD CHOICES

	Portion	Cal	Fat (g)	Sat Fat (g)	Carb (g)	Fiber (g)	Sod (mgs)	Carb Choices	Exchanges
Beef macaroni, Healthy Choice	1 pkg	211	2	0.7	33	4.6	444	2	2 1/2 Starch, 1 1/3 Lean Meat
Beef stew, canned	1 cup	218	12	5.2	16	3.5	947	1	1 Medium-Fat Meat, 3 1/2 Veg, 1 Fat
Chicken pot pie, frozen	1 sm. pie	484	29	9.7	43	1.7	857	3	3 Starch, 1 Lean Meat, 5 Fat
Chili con carne/beans, canned	1 cup	255	8	2.1	24	8.2	1032	1 1/2	1 1/2 Starch, 3 Medium-Fat Meat
Macaroni and cheese, canned	1 cup	199	6	3	29	3	1058	2	1 1/2 Starch, 1 Medium-Fat Meat, 1 Fat
Meatless burger crumbles	1 cup	231	13	3.3	7	5.1	476	1/2	1/2 Starch, 3 Lean Meat, 1 Fat
Meatless burger patty	1 patty	91	1	0.1	8	4.3	383	1/2	1/2 Starch, 1 1/2 Very Lean Meat, 1 Veg
Pasta w/ meatballs, canned	1 cup	260	10	4	31	6.8	1053	2	2 Starch, 1/2 Medium-Fat Meat, 2 Fat
Spaghetti Bolognese, Healthy Choice	1 pkg	255	3	1	43	5.1	473	3	3 Starch, 1/2 Fat

	Portion	Cal	Fat (g)	Sat Fat (g)	Carb (g)	Fiber (g)	Sod (mgs)	Carb Choices	Exchanges
Spaghetti in tomato sauce, canned	1 cup	192	2	0.7	39	7.8	963	2 1/2	2 1/2 Starch
Spinach soufflé, home-made	1 cup	219	18	7.1	3	NA	763	0	1 1/2 Medium-Fat Meat, 1/2 Veg, 3 Fat
Tortellini, cheese filling, cooked	1 cup	249	6	2.9	38	1.5	279	2 1/2	2 1/2 Starch, 1 Lean Meat, 1/3 Fat
Breakfast Items									
Biscuit with egg and sausage	1 biscuit	581	39	15	41	0.9	1141	3	2 1/2 Starch, 1 1/2 Medium-Fat Meat, 6 Fat
Croissant with egg, cheese, bacon	1 croissant	413	28	15.4	24	NA	889	1 1/2	2 Starch, 2 High-Fat Meat, 5 Fat
Danish pastry, cheese-filled	1 pastry	353	25	5.1	29	NA	319	2	2 CHO, 3 1/2 Fat
Danish pastry, fruit-filled	1 pastry	335	16	3.3	45	NA	333	3	3 CHO/ Sugar, 2 3/4 Fat
English muffin w/egg, cheese, and Canadian bacon	1 muffin	289	13	4.7	27	1.5	729	2	2 Starch, 2 Medium-Fat Meat, 1 Fat

	Portion	Cal	Fat (g)	Sat Fat (g)	Carb (g)	Fiber (g)	Sod (mgs)	Carb Choices	Exchanges
French toast with butter	2 slices	356	19	7.7	36	NA	513	2 1/2	2 1/2 Starch, 4 Fat
French toast sticks	5 sticks	513	29	4.7	58	2.7	499	4	4 Starch, 4 Fat
Hashed brown potatoes	1/2 cup	151	9	4.3	16	NA	290	1	1 Starch, 1 1/2 Fat
Pancakes w/butter and syrup	2 pancakes	520	14	5.9	91	NA	1104	6 1/2	5 Starch, 1 CHO/ Sugar, 1 Fat
Burrito with beans and cheese	1	189	6	3.4	27	NA	583	2	2 Starch, 1/2 Medium-Fat Meat, 1 Fat
Burrito with beans and meat	1	255	9	4.2	33	NA	670	2	2 Starch, 1 Fat
Cheeseburger, regular size									
Double patty w/ mayo-type dressing, vegetables	1 sandwich	417	21	8.7	35	NA	1051	2	2 Starch, 2 1/2 Medium-Fat Meat, 3 Fat
Single patty w/ mayo-type dressing, vegetables	1 sandwich	295	14	6.3	27	NA	616	2	2 Starch, 1 Medium-Fat Meat, 1 1/2 Fat
Double patty, plain	1 sandwich	457	28	13	22	NA	636	1 1/2	2 Starch, 2 Medium-Fat Meat, 3 Fat

	Portion	Cal	Fat (g)	Sat Fat (g)	Carb (g)	Fiber (g)	Sod (mgs)	Carb Choices	Exchanges
Double patty, 3-piece bun	1 sandwich	461	22	9.5	44	NA	891	3	3 Starch, 2 Medium-Fat Meat, 2 Fat
Single patty, plain	1 sandwich	319	15	6.5	32	NA	500	2	2 Starch, 2 Medium-Fat Meat, 1 Fat
Cheeseburger, large size									
Single patty w/ mayo-type dressing, vegetables	1 sandwich	563	33	15	38	NA	1108	2 1/2	2 1/2 Starch, 2 Med-Fat Meat, 5 Fat
Single patty with bacon	1 sandwich	608	37	16.2	37	NA	1043	2 1/2	2 1/2 Starch, 3 Medium-Fat Meat, 4 Fat
Chicken Fillet (breaded and fried)	1 sandwich	515	29	8.5	39	NA	957	2 1/2	2 1/2 Starch, 2 1/2 Lean Meat, 4 Fat
Chicken Nuggets, fried	6 pieces	319	21	4.7	15	0	513	1	1 Starch, 2 Medium-Fat Meat, 1 Fat
Chili con carne	1 cup	256	8	3.4	22	NA	1007	1 1/2	1 1/2 Starch, 3 Medium-Fat Meat
Chimichanga with beef	1 piece	425	20	8.5	43	NA	910	3	2 1/2 Starch, 1 1/2 Medium-Fat Meat, 3 Fat

	Portion	Cal	Fat (g)	Sat Fat (g)	Carb (g)	Fiber (g)	Sod (mgs)	Carb Choices	Exchanges
Coleslaw	3/4 cup	147	11	1.6	13	NA	267	1	2 1/2 Veg, 2 Fat
Desserts									
Ice cream, soft, vanilla, w/cone	1 cone	164	6	3.5	24	0.1	92	1 1/2	2 1/2CHO, 1/4 Fat
Pie, fried, with fruit filling	1 pie	404	21	3.1	55	3.3	479	3 1/2	3 1/3 CHO, 4 Fat
Sundae, hot fudge	1 sundae	284	9	5	48	0	182	3	3 CHO, 2 Fat
Enchilada with cheese	1 piece	319	19	10.6	29	NA	784	2	2 Starch, 1/2Medium-Fat Meat, 3 Fat
Fish w/tartar sauce and cheese	1 sandwich	523	29	8.1	48	NA	939	3	3 Starch, 1 1/2 Lean Meat, 4 Fat
French fries	1 small	291	16	3.3	34	3	168	2	2 Starch, 3 Fat
	1 medium	458	25	5.2	53	4.7	265	3 1/2	4 Starch, 4 Fat
	1 large	578	31	6.5	67	5.9	335	4 1/2	4 1/2 Starch, 6 Fat
Frijoles, refried beans, cheese	1 cup	225	8	4.1	29	NA	882	2	3 Starch, 1 Medium-Fat Meat
Hamburger, regular size									
Double patty w/ condiments	1 sandwich	576	32	12	39	NA	742	2 1/2	2 Starch, 3 Medium-Fat Meat, 4 Fat

	Portion	Cal	Fat (g)	Sat Fat (g)	Carb (g)	Fiber (g)	Sod (mgs)	Carb Choices	Exchanges
Single patty w/ condiments	1 sandwich	272	10	3.6	34	2.3	534	2	2 Starch, 1 Medium-Fat Meat, 1 1/2 Fat
Hamburger, large size									
Double patty w/ mayo-type dressing and vegetables	1 sandwich	540	27	10.5	40	NA	791	2 1/2	2 1/2 Starch, 3 Medium-Fat Meat, 3 Fat
Single patty w/ mayo-type dressing and vegetables	1 sandwich	512	27	10.4	40	NA	824	2 1/2	2 1/2 Starch, 2 Medium-Fat Meat, 3 Fat
Hot dog, plain	1 sandwich	242	15	5.1	18	NA	670	1	1 Starch, 1 High-Fat Meat, 2 Fat
Hot dog with chili	1 sandwich	296	13	4.9	31	NA	480	2	1 1/2 Starch, 1 High-Fat Meat, 3 1/2 Fat
Hot dog with corn flour coating	1 corndog	460	19	5.2	56	NA	973	4	4 Starch, 1 High-Fat Meat, 2 1/2 Fat
Hush puppies	5 pieces	257	12	2.7	35	NA	965	2	3 1/2 Starch, 5 Fat
Mashed potatoes	1/3 cup	66	1	0.4	13	NA	182	1	1 Starch

	Portion	Cal	Fat (g)	Sat Fat (g)	Carb (g)	Fiber (g)	Sod (mgs)	Carb Choices	Exchanges
Nachos with cheese sauce	6–8 nachos	346	19	7.8	36	NA	816	2 1/2	2 Starch, 1 High-Fat Meat, 2 Fat
Onion Rings, breaded and fried	8–9 rings	276	16	7	31	NA	430	2	2 Starch, 3 Fat
Pizza (slice = 1/8 of 12" pizza)									
Cheese	1 slice	140	3	1.5	21	NA	336	1 1/2	1 1/4 Starch, 1/2 Medium-Fat Meat, 1/4 Fat
Meat and Vegetables	1 slice	184	5	1.5	21	NA	382	1 1/2	1 1/4 Starch, 1 Medium-Fat Meat, 1/4 Veg
Pepperoni	1 slice	181	7	2.2	20	NA	267	1	1 1/4 Starch, 1 Medium-Fat Meat, 1 Fat
Roast beef sandwich, plain	1 sandwich	346	14	3.6	33	NA	792	2	2 1/4 Starch, 2 Medium-Fat Meat, 1 Fat
Salad, with chicken, no dressing	1 1/2 cups	105	2	0.6	4	NA	209	0	2 Very Lean Meat, 1 1/2 Vegetable
Salad, w/egg, cheese, no dressing	1 1/2 cups	102	6	3	5	NA	119	0	1 Medium-Fat Meat, 1 1/2 Vegetable

	Portion	Cal	Fat (g)	Sat Fat (g)	Carb (g)	Fiber (g)	Sod (mgs)	Carb Choices	Exchanges
Shake, chocolate	16 fl oz	423	12	7.7	68	2.7	323	4 1/2	4 1/2 CHO 2 1/2 Fat
Shake, vanilla	16 fl oz	370	10	6.2	60	1.3	273	4	4 CHO, 2 Fat
Shrimp, breaded and fried	6–8 shrimp	454	25	5.4	40	NA	1446	2 1/2	2 Starch, 2 Very Lean Meat, 4 Fat
Submarine sandwich (6" long)									
Roast beef w/mayo, lettuce and tomato	1 sandwich	410	13	7.1	44	NA	845	3	3 Starch, 2 Medium Fat Meat, 2 Fat
Salami, ham, cheese, w/lettuce, tomato, onion, oil and vinegar	1 sandwich	456	19	6.8	51	NA	1651	3 1/2	3 Starch, 2 High-Fat Meat, 2 Fat
Tuna salad w/mayo and lettuce	1 sandwich	584	28	5.3	55	NA	1293	3 1/2	3 1/2 Starch, 2 1/2 Very Lean Meat, 4 1/2 Fat
Taco, beef, small	1 taco	369	21	11.4	27	NA	802	2	1 1/2 Starch, 2 Medium-Fat Meat, 2 1/2 Fat
Taco, beef, large	1 taco	568	32	17.5	41	NA	1233	3	2 1/2 Starch, 3 1/2 Medium-Fat Meat, 4 Fat

	Portion	Cal	Fat (g)	Sat Fat (g)	Carb (g)	Fiber (g)	Sod (mgs)	Carb Choices	Exchanges
Taco Salad (beef, cheese, taco shell)	1 1/2 cup	279	15	6.8	24	NA	762	1 1/2	1 Starch, 1 Medium-Fat Meat, 1 Veg, 2 Fat
Tostada, beans and beef	1 tostada	333	17	11.5	30	NA	871	2	2 Starch, 1 1/2 Medium-Fat Meat, 2 1/4 Fat
Tostada, with guacamole	1 tostada	181	12	5	16	NA	401	1	1 Starch, 2 Fat

Chapter 24

Brand-Name Convenience Soul Food Choices

From Allen's to Zatarain's, soul food has joined the more than 1,500 varieties of canned foods available. Black-eyed peas, turnip greens, even sweet potato casserole can be found canned or frozen at your local supermarket. Research shows that canned and frozen foods are just as nutritious as fresh and sometimes even better.

Brand-Name Convenience Soul Food Tips:

- ▮●▮ Most canned vegetables are very low in fat or fat-free.

- ▮●▮ Check the Nutrition Facts label to keep sodium low.

- ▮●▮ Rinse canned beans in a strainer under water to reduce some of the sodium content.

- ▮●▮ Many canned foods are available in low-salt and no-salt versions.

- ▮●▮ Canned beans of all types are packed with fiber, protein, and antioxidants.

BRAND-NAME CONVENIENCE SOUL FOOD CHOICES

	Portion	Cal	Fat (g)	Sat Fat (g)	Carb (g)	Fiber (g)	Sod (mgs)	Carb Choices	Exchanges
Allen's Canned Food									
Baked Beans									
Barbeque	1/2 cup	150	1	0	29	5	410	2	2 Starchy Veg
Homestyle	1/2 cup	140	1	0	29	5	410	2	2 Starchy Veg
Maple-Cured Bacon	1/2 cup	140	1	0	27	4	450	2	2 Starchy Veg
Onion	1/2 cup	140	1.5	0	25	4	410	1 1/2	1 1/2 Starchy Veg, 1/3 Fat
Original	1/2 cup	150	1	0	29	8	350	2	2 Starchy Veg
Vegetarian	1/2 cup	140	0	0	28	4	460	2	2 Starchy Veg
Black Beans	1/2 cup	100	0.5	0	19	8	400	1	1 Starchy Veg
Black-eyed peas	1/2 cup	120	1	0	21	6	350	1 1/2	1 1/2 Starchy Veg
Black-eyed peas with Snap	1/2 cup	120	1	0	20	5	420	1	1 Starchy Veg
Black-eyed peas with Bacon	1/2 cup	120	1.5	0.5	20	5	390	1	1 Starchy Veg, 1/3 Fat

	Portion	Cal	Fat (g)	Sat Fat (g)	Carb (g)	Fiber (g)	Sod (mgs)	Carb Choices	Exchanges
Black-eyed peas, dry, soaked	1/2 cup	110	1	0	18	4	275	1	1 Starchy Veg
Butter beans, baby	1/2 cup	120	0.5	0	22	6	460	1 1/2	1 1/2 Starchy Veg
Butter beans, large	1/2 cup	120	1	0	20	7	290	1	1 Starchy Veg
Carrots, tiny, slices	1/2 cup	35	0	0	8	3	40	1/2	1 Veg
Chicken broth	1 cup	10	0	0	0	0	620	0	Free Food
Garbanzo beans	1/2 cup	120	2.5	0	19	8	330	1	1 Starchy Veg, 1/2 Fat
Great northern beans	1/2 cup	100	0.5	0	19	7	310	1	1 Starchy Veg
Green beans									
Cut	1/2 cup	30	0	0	6	3	320	1/2	1 Veg
French style	1/2 cup	25	0	0	4	2	300	0	1 Veg
No salt added	1/2 cup	15	0	0	3	2	10	0	1 Veg
Whole	1/2 cup	30	0	0	6	3	460	1/2	1 Veg
Green bean casserole	1/2 cup	40	1	0	6	1	270	1/2	1 Veg
Greens									
Collard greens, no salt	1/2 cup	30	0.5	0	5	3	20	0	1 Veg
Collard greens, seasoned	1/2 cup	35	0.5	0	5	1	830	0	1 Veg

	Portion	Cal	Fat (g)	Sat Fat (g)	Carb (g)	Fiber (g)	Sod (mgs)	Carb Choices	Exchanges
Kale greens, no salt	1/2 cup	30	0.5	0	3	2	20	0	1 Veg
Kale greens, seasoned	1/2 cup	35	0.5	0	5	1	830	0	1 Veg
Mixed greens, no salt	1/2 cup	30	0.5	0	8	4	10	1/2	1 Veg
Mixed greens, seasoned	1/2 cup	45	0.5	0	6	1	830	1/2	1 Veg
Mustard greens, no salt	1/2 cup	30	0.5	0	5	3	10	0	1 Veg
Mustard greens, seasoned	1/2 cup	45	0.5	0	6	1	830	1/2	1 Veg
Turnip greens, no salt	1/2 cup	25	0.5	0	3	2	15	0	1 Veg
Turnip greens, seasoned	1/2 cup	35	0.5	0	5	2	860	0	1 Veg
Turnip greens and turnips, no salt	1/2 cup	30	0.5	0	5	3	20	0	1 Veg
Turnip greens and turnips, seasoned	1/2 cup	35	0.5	0	5	2	860	0	1 Veg
Hominy									
Golden	1/2 cup	120	0.5	0	27	4	340	2	2 Starchy Veg

	Portion	Cal	Fat (g)	Sat Fat (g)	Carb (g)	Fiber (g)	Sod (mgs)	Carb Choices	Exchanges
Pepi golden	1/2 cup	120	0.5	0	27	4	340	2	2 Starchy Veg
White	1/2 cup	100	0.5	0	22	4	340	1 1/2	1 1/2 Starchy Veg
Italian green beans, cut	1/2 cup	35	0	0	7	3	320	1/2	1 Veg
Italian green beans, seasoned	1/2 cup	45	0	0	8	3	370	1/2	1 Veg
Italian green beans, shellouts	1/2 cup	50	0	0	9	3	320	1/2	1 Veg
Italian green beans w/ potatoes	1/2 cup	50	0	0	10	2	160	1/2	1 Veg
Kidney beans, dark red	1/2 cup	130	0.5	0	22	8	310	1 1/2	1 1/2 Starchy Veg
Kidney beans, light red	1/2 cup	120	0.5	0	22	8	340	1 1/2	1 1/2 Starchy Veg
Lima beans, green and white	1/2 cup	110	1	0	20	9	280	1	1 Starchy Veg
Lima beans, medium green	1/2 cup	120	0	0	23	8	370	1 1/2	1 1/2 Starchy Veg
Navy beans	1/2 cup	110	1	0	19	6	380	1	1 Starchy Veg
Okra, cut	1/2 cup	30	0	0	6	3	400	1/2	1 Veg
Okra and tomatoes, cut	1/2 cup	30	0	0	5	3	380	0	1 Veg
Okra, tomatoes, and corn, cut	1/2 cup	30	0	0	6	4	280	1/2	1 Veg

	Portion	Cal	Fat (g)	Sat Fat (g)	Carb (g)	Fiber (g)	Sod (mgs)	Carb Choices	Exchanges
Peas									
Crowder	1/2 cup	110	1	0	19	8	460	1	1 Starchy Veg
Field peas w/snaps	1/2 cup	120	1	0	21	6	300	1 1/2	1 1/2 Starchy Veg
Purple hull	1/2 cup	120	1	0	21	6	350	1 1/2	1 1/2 Starchy Veg
Pinto beans	1/2 cup	110	1	0	20	7	290	1	1 Starchy Veg
Princella yams, cut, in syrup	1/2 cup	90	<1	0	20	2	28	1	1 Starchy Veg
Princella yams, cut, in water	1/2 cup	80	<1	0	16	2	25	1	1 Starchy Veg
Princella yams, mashed	1/2 cup	100	<1	0	24	3	45	1 1/2	1 1/2 Starchy Veg
Red beans	1/2 cup	100	0.5	0	19	9	310	1	1 Starchy Veg
Refried beans	1/2 cup	150	2.5	1	24	11	360	1 1/2	1 1/2 Starchy Veg, 1/2 Fat
Refried beans, no fat added	1/2 cup	120	0	0	23	8	500	1 1/2	1 Starchy Veg
Royal Prince yams									
Orange-pineapple	1/2 cup	180	<1	0	35	2	60	2	1 Starchy Veg, 1 CHO
Whole in light syrup	1/2 cup	110	<1	0	24	2	30	1 1/2	1 Starchy Veg, 1/2 CHO

	Portion	Cal	Fat (g)	Sat Fat (g)	Carb (g)	Fiber (g)	Sod (mgs)	Carb Choices	Exchanges
Whole in heavy syrup	1/2 cup	120	<1	0	26	2	32	2	1 Starchy Veg, 1 CHO
Bruce's Canned Food									
Okra, cut	1/2 cup	18	0.1	0	4	2	415	0	1 Veg
Okra and tomatoes	1/2 cup	14	0.1	0	3	1	206	0	1 Veg
Okra, tomatoes, and corn	1/2 cup	15	0.1	0	3	1	191	0	1 Veg
Squash, yellow	1/2 cup	15	0.1	0	3	<1	177	0	1 Veg
Yams									
Candied	1/2 cup	120	0.2	0	29	1.2	111	2	2 Starchy Veg
Mashed	1/2 cup	86	0.4	0	19	2	26	1	1 Starchy Veg
Whole	1/2 cup	122	0.2	0	29	2	13	2	2 Starchy Veg
w/Orange-pineapple sauce	1/2 cup	115	0.3	0	27	2	13	2	2 Starchy Veg
Whole, vacuum-packed	1/2 cup	84	0.3	0	19	3	10	1	1 Starchy Veg
East Texas Fair Canned Food									
Black-eyed peas	1/2 cup	120	1	0	21	6	350	1 1/2	1 1/2 Starchy Veg

	Portion	Cal	Fat (g)	Sat Fat (g)	Carb (g)	Fiber (g)	Sod (mgs)	Carb Choices	Exchanges
Black-eyed peas w/snaps	1/2 cup	120	1	0	20	5	420	1	1 Starchy Veg
Chick peas	1/2 cup	120	2.5	0	19	8	330	1	1 Starchy Veg
Lima beans, green	1/2 cup	120	0	0	23	8	370	1 1/2	1 1/2 Starchy Veg
Peas									
Crowder	1/2 cup	110	1	0	19	8	460	1	1 Starchy Veg
Cream	1/2 cup	100	1	0	17	5	460	1	1 Starchy Veg
Field peas w/snaps	1/2 cup	120	1	0	21	6	300	1 1/2	1 1/2 Starchy Veg
Jalapeño pepper	1/2 cup	120	1	0	22	6	580	1 1/2	1 1/2 Starchy Veg
Peas and pork	1/2 cup	110	1.5	0.5	19	5	540	1	1 Starchy Veg
Purple hull	1/2 cup	120	1	0	21	6	350	1 1/2	1 1/2 Starchy Veg
White acre peas	1/2 cup	100	1	0	17	5	460	1	1 Starchy Veg
Glory Canned Foods									
Black beans and rice	1/2 cup	90	1.5	0	16	2	450	1	1 Starch
Black-eyed peas	1/2 cup	140	0.5	0	25	5	420	1 1/2	1 1/2 Starch

	Portion	Cal	Fat (g)	Sat Fat (g)	Carb (g)	Fiber (g)	Sod (mgs)	Carb Choices	Exchanges
Black-eyed peas and rice	1/2 cup	90	0.5	0	17	3	680	1	1 Starch
Butter beans	1/2 cup	120	1	0.5	20	5	530	1	1 Starch
Candied yams	1/2 cup	210	0	0	52	1	240	3 1/2	3 1/2 Starchy Veg
Collard greens	1/2 cup	50	1	0	7	3	470	1/2	1 Veg
Country cabbage	1/2 cup	30	0	0	6	2	300	1/2	1 Veg
Creamed peas	1/2 cup	80	1	0.5	13	3	530	1	1 Starchy Veg
Crock pot beans	1/2 cup	130	0.5	0	25	7	610	1 1/2	1 1/2 Starch
Field beans	1/2 cup	80	0	0	14	4	830	1	1 Starch
Field peas with snaps	1/2 cup	70	0	0	12	5	830	1	1 Starchy Veg
Fried apples	1/2 cup	80	0	0	21	1	170	1 1/2	1 Fruit, 1/2 Fat
Great northern beans	1/2 cup	90	0.5	0	15	3	850	1	1 Starchy Veg
Green bean casserole	1/2 cup	45	0.5	0	9	2	480	1/2	1 Veg
Honey carrots	1/2 cup	50	0	0	13	2	220	1	1 Veg
Hot sauce	1 tsp	0	0	0	0	0	130	0	Free Food
Kale greens	1/2 cup	50	0.5	0	6	3	440	1/2	1 Veg
Lima beans	1/2 cup	140	1	0.5	24	7	620	1 1/2	1 1/2 Starchy Veg
Mixed greens	1/2 cup	50	0.5	0	7	3	470	1/2	1 Veg
Mustard greens	1/2 cup	50	0.5	0	7	3	460	1/2	1 Veg

	Portion	Cal	Fat (g)	Sat Fat (g)	Carb (g)	Fiber (g)	Sod (mgs)	Carb Choices	Exchanges
New Orleans-style red beans	1/2 cup	130	0	0	22	7	680	1 1/2	1 1/2 Starchy Veg
Okra	1/2 cup	25	0	0	6	2	0	1/2	1 Veg
Pinto beans	1/2 cup	90	0.5	0	15	5	850	1	1 Starchy Veg
Pole beans	1/2 cup	45	0	0	9	2	430	1/2	1 Veg
Red beans and rice	1/2 cup	90	0.5	0	18	3	680	1	1 Starch
Scalloped potatoes	1/2 cup	70	0.5	0	14	1	590	1	1 Starchy Veg
Skillet corn	1/2 cup	90	0.5	0	22	2	580	1 1/2	1 Starchy Veg
Smothered potatoes									
With herbs and garlic	1/2 cup	50	0	0	11	1	540	1	1 Starchy Veg
With beef gravy	1/2 cup	50	0	0	11	<1	600	1	1 Starchy Veg
With chicken gravy	1/2 cup	50	0	0	11	<1	820	1	1 Starchy Veg
Spinach	1/2 cup	30	0	0	3	2	430	0	1 Veg
String beans	1/2 cup	30	0.5	0	6	2	410	1/2	1 Veg
String beans w/potatoes	1/2 cup	50	0.5	0	10	2	580	1/2	1 Veg, 1/4 Starchy Veg
Succotash	1/2 cup	80	0	0	17	3	580	1	1 Starchy Veg
Sweet potatoes	1/2 cup	120	0	0	30	2	30	2	1 Starchy Veg, 1/2 CHO/ Sugar

	Portion	Cal	Fat (g)	Sat Fat (g)	Carb (g)	Fiber (g)	Sod (mgs)	Carb Choices	Exchanges
Sweet potato casserole	1/2 cup	180	0	0	43	2	250	3	1 Starchy Veg, 1 CHO/ Sugar
Turkey-flavored collard greens	1/2 cup	40	0.5	0	6	2	510	1/2	1 Veg
Turkey-flavored turnip greens	1/2 cup	35	0	0	5	2	540	0	1 Veg
Turnip greens	1/2 cup	45	0.5	0	6	2	630	1/2	1 Veg
Turnip greens w/diced turnips	1/2 cup	35	0	0	6	2	430	1/2	1 Veg
Luck's Canned Foods									
Black-eyed peas									
Fat-free	1/2 cup	100	0	0	18	3	400	1	1 Starchy Veg
Seasoned with pork	1/2 cup	120	2	0.5	20	4	350	1	1 Starchy Veg
Great northern beans									
Fat-free	1/2 cup	110	0	0	20	6	400	1	1 Starchy Veg
Seasoned with pork	1/2 cup	120	2	0.5	20	6	370	1	1 Starchy Veg
Pinto beans, seasoned w/ pork	1/2 cup	130	2	0.5	22	6	410	1 1/2	1 1/2 Starchy Veg

	Portion	Cal	Fat (g)	Sat Fat (g)	Carb (g)	Fiber (g)	Sod (mgs)	Carb Choices	Exchanges
Margaret Holmes									
Peaches									
Greer southern freestone	1/2 cup	100	0	0	25	2	770	1 1/2	1 1/2 Fruit
O'sage lite raggedy ripe freestone	1/2 cup	70	0	0	19	1	0	1	1 Fruit
Sunshine spiced whole pickled	1 peach	70	0	0	16	0	5	1	1 Fruit
Peanuts									
Cajun-style boiled peanuts	2 Tbsp	100	8	1.5	3	2	320	0	2 Fat
Green boiled peanuts, canned	2 Tbsp	100	8	1.5	3	2	390	0	2 Fat
Green boiled peanuts, pouched	1/4 cup	110	7	1	7	0	250	1/2	1 1/2 Fat
Ready Recipes									
Black-eyed peas and rice	1 cup	160	2	0	33	3	1080	2	2 Starch
Green bean casserole	1/2 cup	50	2	0	8	2	420	1/2	1 Veg, 1/2 Fat
Jambalaya	1 cup	160	2.5	0	34	1	1150	2	2 Starch, 1/2 Fat
Potato casserole	1/2 cup	100	4	1	16	2	430	1	1 Starch, 1 Fat
Red beans and rice	1 cup	190	3	0.5	42	7	950	3	2 1/2 Starch

	Portion	Cal	Fat (g)	Sat Fat (g)	Carb (g)	Fiber (g)	Sod (mgs)	Carb Choices	Exchanges
Squash casserole	1 cup	100	4	1	19	5	1000	1	1 Starch, 1 Fat
Seasoned Southern Classics									
Seasoned black-eyed peas	1/2 cup	120	0.5	0	26	6	790	2	1 1/2 Starchy Veg
Seasoned butter beans	1/2 cup	110	1.5	0	21	5	770	1 1/2	1 1/2 Starchy Veg
Seasoned cabbage	1/2 cup	30	0	0	6	2	300	1/2	1 Veg
Seasoned collard greens	1/2 cup	35	1.5	0	7	3	390	1/2	1 Veg
Seasoned field peas and snaps	1/2 cup	130	0.5	0	25	8	790	1 1/2	1 1/2 Starchy Veg
Seasoned mixed greens	1/2 cup	35	1.5	0	16	3	390	1	1 Veg
Seasoned turnip greens	1/2 cup	35	1.5	0	7	3	390	1/2	1 Veg
Seasoned turnip greens and roots	1/2 cup	35	1.5	0	7	3	390	1/2	1 Veg
Southern Classics									
Butter peas	1/2 cup	130	0	0	24	4	240	1 1/2	1 1/2 Starchy Veg
Cut okra	1/2 cup	25	0	0	6	2	180	1/2	1 Veg

	Portion	Cal	Fat (g)	Sat Fat (g)	Carb (g)	Fiber (g)	Sod (mgs)	Carb Choices	Exchanges
Diced rutabagas	1/2 cup	35	0	0	6	2	300	1/2	1 Veg
Hoppin' John	1/2 cup	80	0	0	16	4	321	1	1 Starch
Seasoned rutabagas	1/2 cup	35	0	0	6	2	300	1/2	1 Veg
Squash	1/2 cup	25	0	0	5	2	300	0	1 Veg
Squash with Vidalia onions	1/2 cup	25	0	0	6	2	300	1/2	1 Veg
Tomatoes and okra	1/2 cup	30	0	0	7	1	326	1/2	1 Veg
Tomatoes, okra, and corn	1/2 cup	45	0	0	10	1	326	1/2	1 Veg
Triple succotash	1/2 cup	60	0	0	13	2	326	1	1 Starchy Veg
McKenzie's									
Baby lima beans	1/2 cup	110	0.5	0	22	5	140	1 1/2	1 1/2 Starchy Veg
Field peas	1/2 cup	110	0.5	0	21	4	10	1 1/2	1 1/2 Starchy Veg
Fruit, frozen	1 cup	60	0	0	13	2	20	1	1 Fruit
Garden fresh mixtures	1/2 cup	25	0	0	4	2	25	0	1 Veg
Gold king breaded okra	1/2 cup	90	0.5	0	NA	NA	350	NA	NA
Okra, cut	1/2 cup	25	0	0	5	3	35	0	1 Veg
Okra, tomatoes w/ onions	1/2 cup	20	0	0	4	2	30	0	1 Veg
Pole beans, cut	1/2 cup	25	0	0	4	2	10	0	1 Veg

	Portion	Cal	Fat (g)	Sat Fat (g)	Carb (g)	Fiber (g)	Sod (mgs)	Carb Choices	Exchanges
Purple hull peas	1/2 cup	110	0.5	0	21	4	10	1 1/2	1 1/2 Starch
Southern white corn	1/2 cup	80	1	0	19	1	10	1	1 Starchy Veg
Speckled butter beans	1/2 cup	100	0	0	20	4	130	1	1 1/4 Starchy Veg
Vegetable gumbo mixture	1 cup	35	0	0	8	2	30	1/2	1 Veg
Vegetable soup mix	1 cup	40	0	0	9	2	40	1/2	1 Veg
Whole okra	1/2 cup	25	0	0	5	3	35	0	1 Veg
Sylvia's Soul foods									
Greens and Yams									
Seasoned collard greens	1/2 cup	45	1	0	8	3	475	1/2	1 Veg, 1/4 Fat
Seasoned mixed greens	1/2 cup	45	1.5	0	7	2	590	1/2	1 Veg, 1/3 Fat
Seasoned mustard greens	1/2 cup	45	1	0	7	2	475	1/2	1 Veg, 1/4 Fat
Seasoned turnip greens	1/2 cup	40	1	0	7	2	475	1/2	1 Veg, 1/4 Fat
Yams in light syrup	1/2 cup	120	0	0	30	2	30	2	2 Starchy Veg
Miscellaneous Mixes									
Brown gravy mix	1/4 cup	20	0	0	4	0	280	0	1/4 Starch

	Portion	Cal	Fat (g)	Sat Fat (g)	Carb (g)	Fiber (g)	Sod (mgs)	Carb Choices	Exchanges
Chicken gravy mix	1/4 cup	20	0.5	0	4	0	250	0	1/4 Starch
Country gravy mix	1/4 cup	50	2.5	0.5	5	0	290	0	1/4 Starch, 1/2 Fat
Crisp fried chicken mix	1 Tbsp	30	0	0	6	0	460	1/2	1/2 Starch
Fish fry mix	3 Tbsp	100	1	0	20	0	710	1	1 1/4 Starch
Flapjack and pancake mix	1/3 cup	190	4	1	35	0	820	2	2 1/2 Starch, 1 Fat
Golden corn bread and muffin mix	1/4 cup	160	4.5	1	29	0	290	2	2 Starch, 1 Fat
Hush puppies mix	1/3 cup	130	2	0	24	0	500	1 1/2	1 1/2 Starch, 1/2 Fat
Peach cobbler mix	1/4 cup	150	0	0	35	0	140	2	2 1/2 Starch
Peas and Beans									
Seasoned baby lima beans	1/2 cup	110	2.5	1	18	4	690	1	1 Starchy Veg, 1/2 Fat
Seasoned black-eyed peas	1/2 cup	110	3	0.5	15	3	475	1	1 Starchy Veg, 1/2 Fat
Seasoned field peas with snaps	1/2 cup	120	3.5	0.5	17	3	475	1	1 Starchy Veg, 3/4 Fat
Seasoned kidney beans	1/2 cup	110	3	0.5	15	4	475	1	1 Starchy Veg, 1/2 Fat

	Portion	Cal	Fat (g)	Sat Fat (g)	Carb (g)	Fiber (g)	Sod (mgs)	Carb Choices	Exchanges
Seasoned pinto beans	1/2 cup	120	3	0.5	17	5	475	1	1 Starchy Veg, 1/2 Fat
Sauces									
Honey mustard sweet and tangy	1 Tbsp	5	0	0	1	0	70	0	Free Food
Kicking hot, hot	1 tsp	0	0	0	0	0	130	0	Free Food
Original—hot and sassy	2 Tbsp	35	0	0	8	1	280	1/2	1/2 Starch
Original— mild and tangy	2 Tbsp	40	0	0	9	1	290	1/2	1/2 Starch
Smokin' soul BBQ—mild	2 Tbsp	25	0	0	6	0	220	1/2	1/2 Starch
Smokin' soul BBQ—spicy hot	2 Tbsp	25	0	0	6	0	220	1/2	1/2 Starch
Soulful house dressing	2 Tbsp	100	8	1	6	0	170	1/2	1/2 Starch, 1 1/2 Fat
Triple strength hot	1 tsp	0	0	0	0	0	120	0	Free Food
Soups									
Black-eyed pea soup	1 cup	180	2	0	32	6	740	2	2 Starchy Veg, 1/2 Fat
Navy bean soup	1 cup	170	1.5	0	29	9	800	2	2 Starchy Veg, 1/3 Fat
Spices and Seasonings									
Garlic salt	1/4 tsp	0	0	0	0	0	180	0	Free Food

	Portion	Cal	Fat (g)	Sat Fat (g)	Carb (g)	Fiber (g)	Sod (mgs)	Carb Choices	Exchanges
Hot spice sizzlin' seasoning	1/4 tsp	0	0	0	0	0	280	0	Free Food
Lemon pepper	1/4 tsp	0	0	0	0	0	180	0	Free Food
Pure black pepper	1/4 tsp	0	0	0	0	0	0	0	Free Food
Pure garlic powder	1/4 tsp	0	0	0	0	0	0	0	Free Food
Soulful seasoned salt	1/4 tsp	0	0	0	0	0	320	0	Free Food
Zatarain's									
Corn bread stuffing mix	1/4 cup	100	1	0	21	0	320	1 1/2	1 1/2 Starch
Crab cake mix	4 Tbsp	100	0.5	0	24	0	410	1 1/2	1 1/2 Starch
Creole chicken stuffing, prepared	1/2 cup	100	1	0	20	1	530	1	1 1/4 Starch
Fish-fry, seasoned bread mix	1 1/2 Tbsp	40	0	0	9	0	510	1/2	3/4 Starch
Hush puppy mix	3 Tbsp	100	0.5	0	23	<1	320	1 1/2	1 1/2 Starch
New Orleans Style									
Chicken creole mix, prepared	1 cup	130	1	0	28	0	690	2	2 Starch
Dirty brown rice mix, prepared	1 cup	150	1.5	0	31	1	660	2	2 Starch
Étouffée base prepared	1 cup	35	0	0	7	0	380	1/2	1/2 Starch

	Portion	Cal	Fat (g)	Sat Fat (g)	Carb (g)	Fiber (g)	Sod (mgs)	Carb Choices	Exchanges
Gumbo base prepared	1 cup	45	0	0	9	0	620	1/2	1/2 Starch
Gumbo mix w/rice, prepared	1 cup	70	0	0	16	0	630	1	1 Starch
Jambalaya mix, prepared	1 cup	130	0	0	29	0	460	2	2 Starch
Shrimp Creole base, prepared	1 cup	20	0	0	4	0	460	0	Free Food
Red beans and rice, prepared	1 cup	180	0.5	0	41	4	970	3	3 Starch
Red beans seasoning, prepared	1/2 cup	10	0	0	2	0	290	0	Free Food
Red beans, rice, and sausage, frozen	1 entrée	560	20	7	76	10	1190	5	5 Starch, 4 Fat
Red beans, rice, and sausage, frozen	1 cup	373	13	5	51	7	793	3 1/2	3 1/2 Starch, 2 1/2 Fat

Chapter 25

Eating Soulfully and Healthfully for Life

Changing your eating habits can be the most challenging aspect of diabetes self-management. It requires hard work, practice, and discipline. Every day you will need to make choices that will affect your diabetes and your life.

Now that you've read this book, you are prepared to make healthy choices. However, *Eating Soulfully and Healthfully with Diabetes* is not the kind of book that you read once and put back on the shelf. You will refer to this book often as you plan your meals and manage your diabetes.

In Appendix A, you will find sample menus. Many people find it easier to follow sample menus when newly diagnosed with diabetes. There is no doubt that when you read the menus, you will find foods that don't appeal to your appetite. If you don't eat a particular food on the menu, simply substitute a food of similar value. Think of the menu as a road map to daily meal planning.

Appendix B provides a sample food diary to help you put it all together. You can record your daily food choices, carbohydrate counts, and blood glucose levels in the diary. The information you gather can be especially helpful when you want to determine the effect your food has on your blood glucose levels. Take your diary with you when you go to your doctor or diabetes educator. The information from your food diary will help your health-care provider manage your diabetes.

Also, when visiting your doctor, dietitian, or diabetes educator, use the Soul Food Dictionary in Appendix C to shorten the cultural distance between you and your health-care team. Help them to understand how you incorporate certain foods into your meal plan.

Finally, as you continue to manage your diabetes and eat soulfully and healthfully for life, remember these healthful tips:

♦ Eat the right portions of healthy food, such as fruits and vegetables, fish, lean meats, dry beans, whole grains, and low-fat or skim milk and cheese.

♦ Eat foods that have less salt and fat.

♦ Do not add salt to your food after it is cooked.

♦ stay at a healthy weight by being active and eating the right amounts of healthy foods.

♦ Get 30–60 minutes of activity on most days of the week.

♦ Check your blood glucose the way your doctor tells you to.

♦ Take medications the way your doctor tells you.

♦ Stop smoking; seek help to quit.

♦ Check your feet every day for cuts, blisters, red spots, and swelling. Call your health-care team right away about any sores that won't heal.

♦ Brush your teeth and floss every day to avoid problems with your mouth, teeth, or gums.

♦ See your health-care team at least twice a year to find and treat problems early.

Remember, you can eat soulfully and healthfully with diabetes!

Appendix A

Seven-Day Soul Food Menus

45–60 g carbohydrates per meal

Day 1

Breakfast

	Total Carbohydrate (g)
3/4 c. Cheerios®	15
1 c. skim milk	12
1 small banana (4 oz)	30
coffee/tea with artificial sweetener	0
TOTAL	**57**

Lunch

1 slice of pizza (of 8-slice pie)	
dough	30
1 oz. mozzarella cheese	0
1/2 c. tomato sauce	0
mixed salad	
1 c. romaine lettuce	5
1/2 c. sliced tomatoes	3
1 tbsp. Italian salad dressing	0
1 c. honeydew melon cubes	15
calorie-free beverage	0
TOTAL	**53**

Dinner

1 baked salmon croquette (4 oz.)	
1/4 c. breadcrumbs	15
3 oz. salmon	0
1 tsp. margarine	0
1/2 c. boiled potatoes with parsley garnish	15
1/2 c. cooked mustard greens	5
1 piece cornbread (2" square)	15
1 tsp. margarine	0
1/2 mango (5 1/2 oz)	15
calorie-free beverage	0
TOTAL	**65**

Snack

6 saltine crackers	15
2 tsp. peanut butter	0
calorie-free beverage	0
TOTAL	**15**

Day 2

Breakfast

	Total Carbohydrate (g)
1 c. oatmeal	30
1/2 c. skim milk	6
1/4 c. blueberries	5
1 slice whole-wheat toast	15
1 tsp. margarine	0
coffee/tea with artificial sweetener	0
TOTAL	**56**

Lunch

1 small multi-grain roll (2 oz.)	30
3 oz. shredded cooked lean pork	0
1 tbsp. barbeque sauce	15
1/3 c. baked beans	15
cucumber salad	
1 c. cucumber slices	5
1 tbsp. vinaigrette salad dressing	0
1 c. sugar-free Jell-o®	0
calorie-free beverage	0
TOTAL	**65**

Dinner

4 oz. lean boneless broiled sirloin steak	0
1/2 cup sautéed mushrooms and onions	5
2 tsp. canola oil	0
1 small baked potato (3 oz.)	15
2 tbsp. low-fat sour cream	0
1/2 c. cooked broccoli	5
1 tsp. margarine	0
1/2 c. bread pudding	
1 slice white bread	15
1/2 c. skim milk	6
1/8 c. raisins	2
artificial sweetener	0
1 tbsp. Cool Whip® topping	0
calorie-free beverage	0
TOTAL	**48**

Snack

3/4 c. sugar-free cherry yogurt	15
calorie-free beverage	0
TOTAL	**15**

Day 3

Breakfast	Total Carbohydrate (g)
1/4 c. scrambled Egg Beaters	0
1 toasted whole-wheat English muffin	30
1 tsp. margarine	0
2 tsp. sugar-free jelly	0
3/4 c. pineapple cubes (in own juice)	15
coffee/tea with artificial sweetener	0
2 tbsp. skim milk in coffee/tea	0
TOTAL	**45**

Lunch

2 slices seven-grain bread	30
1/2 c. tuna fish (canned in water)	0
1 tbsp. reduced-fat mayonnaise	0
2 lettuce leaves	0
2 slices onion	0
1 1/4 c. watermelon	15
calorie-free beverage	0
TOTAL	**45**

Dinner

smothered pork chop	
4 oz. broiled pork chop (trim off fat)	0
1/4 c. defatted gravy	7
Hoppin' John	
1/2 c. cooked black-eyed peas	15
1/2 c. steamed white rice	20
1/2 c. cooked collard greens (no fat)	5
1 tsp. margarine	0
baked apple	
1 small baked apple (4 oz)	15
1 tsp. ground cinnamon	0
artificial sweetener	0
calorie-free beverage	0
TOTAL	**62**

Snack

finger sndwiches	
6 Triscuit® crackers	15
1 oz. cooked turkey (white meat)	0
calorie-free beverage	0
TOTAL	**15**

Day 4

Breakfast	Total Carbohydrate (g)
3 oz. turkey sausage patty	0
1/2 oz. low-fat cheddar cheese	0
1 small Lender's® bagel (2 oz)	30
1 small orange (6–1/2 oz)	15
coffee/tea with artificial sweetener	0
2 tbsp. skim milk in coffee/tea	0
TOTAL	**45**

Lunch

1 c. chicken gumbo soup	
1 c. chicken broth	0
2 oz. broiled skinless chicken	0
1/2 c. cooked corn, onion, and okra	15
1 whole-wheat deli roll (1 oz)	15
tossed salad	
1 c. romaine and iceberg lettuce mix	5
1/4 c. chopped tomato	0
1/2 c. low-fat croutons	7
1 tbsp. French dressing	0
1 medium peach (6 oz)	15
calorie-free beverage	0
TOTAL	**57**

Dinner

4 oz. roasted turkey (white meat, without skin)	0
1/2 c. mashed potatoes	15
1/4 c. milk in mashed potatoes	3
1/2 c. cooked green beans	5
1 tsp. margarine	0
1/2 cup cranberries	15
1/2 c. corn bread dressing	15
calorie-free beverage	0
TOTAL	**53**

Snack

trail mix	
3/4 oz. pretzels	15
10 peanuts	0
calorie-free beverage	0
TOTAL	**15**

Day 5

Breakfast	Total Carbohydrate (g)
1 medium corn muffin (2 oz.)	30
1 tsp. margarine	0
1/2 c. low-fat cottage cheese	3
1/2 c. canned peaches (in own juice)	15
coffee/tea with artificial sweetener	0
2 tbsp. skim milk in coffee/tea	0
TOTAL	**48**

Lunch

3 oz. grilled turkey burger	0
1 oz. low-fat cheddar cheese	0
1 whole-wheat bun (2 oz.)	30
1 cup cole slaw (prepared with low-fat mayo)	5
1 medium pear (4 oz.)	30
calorie-free beverage	0
TOTAL	**65**

Dinner

chicken and dumplings	
4 oz baked chicken (remove all skin)	0
2 dumplings (2"x 2" each)	30
1/4 c. defatted gravy	7
1/2 c. cooked carrots	5
1 tsp. margarine	0
1/2 c. sugar-free frozen yogurt	15
calorie-free beverage	0
TOTAL	**57**

Snack

3 graham crackers (2 1/2" square)	15
1/2 c. skim milk	6
calorie-free beverage	0
TOTAL	**21**

Day 6

Breakfast	Total Carbohydrate (g)
western omelet	
3 scrambled egg whites	0
1/2 c. cooked green peppers and onions	5
1/2 c. cooked grits	15
1 small biscuit (2 1/2" across)	15
1 tsp. margarine	0
17 small grapes (3 oz)	15
coffee/tea with artificial sweetener	0
2 tbsp. skim milk in coffee/tea	0
TOTAL	**50**

Lunch

2 slices rye bread	30
3 oz. sliced cooked roast beef	0
1 tsp. mayonnaise	0
1/2 cup potato salad (made with low-fat mayo)	15
1/2 c. fruit cocktail (in own juice)	15
calorie-free beverage	0
TOTAL	**60**

Dinner

4 oz. baked fresh lean ham	0
1 small baked sweet potato (3 oz)	15
1/2 c. cooked turnip greens	5
1 small biscuit (2 1/2" across)	15
1 tsp. margarine	0
1/2 c. unsweetened applesauce	15
calorie-free beverage	0
TOTAL	**50**

Snack

nachos	
9 baked tortilla chips (1 oz)	15
1 oz. low-fat cheddar cheese	0
1/4 c. salsa	0
calorie-free beverage	0
TOTAL	**15**

Day 7

Breakfast	Total Carbohydrate (g)
2 pancakes (4" across)	15
2 tbsp. sugar-free maple syrup	0
3/4 c. vanilla low-fat yogurt	12
1 1/4 c. whole strawberries	15
coffee/tea with artificial sweetener	0
2 tbsp. skim milk in coffee/tea	0
TOTAL	**42**

Lunch

1 c. chili	
3 oz lean pan-broiled ground beef	0
1/2 c. tomato sauce	5
1/4 c. cooked green peppers	2
1/4 c. cooked onions	2
1/2 c. cooked kidney beans	15
1/3 c. steamed white rice	15
1/2 c. sugar-free vanilla ice cream	15
calorie-free beverage	0
TOTAL	**54**

Dinner

4 oz. blackened catfish	0
stewed tomatoes and okra	
1/2 c. cooked okra	5
1/4 c. stewed tomatoes	3
1/2 c. steamed brown rice	20
1 small biscuit (2 1/2" across)	15
1 tsp. margarine	0
1 c. cantaloupe melon cubes	15
calorie-free beverage	0
TOTAL	**58**

Snack

1 c. sugar-free pudding (made with skim milk)	12
calorie-free beverage	0
TOTAL	**12**

Seven-Day Soul Food Menus: 60–75 g carbohydrates per meal

Day 1

Breakfast	Total Carbohydrate (g)
1 1/2 c. Cheerios®	30
1 c. skim milk	12
1 small banana (4 oz)	30
coffee/tea with artificial sweetener	0
TOTAL	**72**

Lunch
1 slice of pizza (of 8-slice pie)	
dough	30
1 oz. mozzarella cheese	0
1/4 c. tomato sauce	0
mixed salad	
2 c. romaine lettuce	5
1 c. sliced tomatoes	6
1 tbsp. Italian salad dressing	0
2 c. honeydew melon cubes	30
calorie-free beverage	0
TOTAL	**71**

Dinner
1 baked salmon croquette (4 oz.)	
¼ c. breadcrumbs	15
3 oz. salmon	0
1 tsp. margarine	0
1/2 c. boiled potatoes with parsley garnish	15
1 1/2 c. cooked mustard greens	15
1 piece cornbread (2" square)	15
1 tsp. margarine	0
1/2 mango (5 1/2 oz)	15
calorie-free beverage	0
TOTAL	**75**

Snack
6 saltine crackers	15
2 tsp. peanut butter	0
calorie-free beverage	0
TOTAL	**15**

Day 2

Breakfast	Total Carbohydrate (g)
1 c. oatmeal	30
1/2 c. skim milk	6
1/4 c. blueberries	5
2 slices whole-wheat toast	30
1 tsp. margarine	0
coffee/tea with artificial sweetener	0
TOTAL	**71**

Lunch
1 small multi-grain roll (2 oz.)	30
3 oz. shredded cooked lean pork	0
1 tbsp. barbeque sauce	15
1/2 c. baked beans	23
cucumber salad	
1 c. cucumber slices	5
1 tbsp. vinaigrette salad dressing	0
1 c. sugar-free Jell-o®	0
calorie-free beverage	0
TOTAL	**73**

Dinner
4 oz. lean boneless broiled sirloin steak	0
1/2 cup sautéed mushrooms and onions	5
2 tsp. canola oil	0
1 medium baked potato (6 oz.)	30
2 Tbsp. low-fat sour cream	0
1/2 c. cooked broccoli	5
1 tsp. margarine	0
1/2 c. bread pudding	
1 slice white bread	15
1/2 c. skim milk	6
1/8 c. raisins	2
artificial sweetener	0
1 tbsp. Cool Whip® topping	0
calorie-free beverage	0
TOTAL	**73**

Snack
3/4 c. sugar-free cherry yogurt	15
calorie-free beverage	0
TOTAL	**15**

Day 3

Breakfast	Total Carbohydrate (g)
1/2 c. scrambled Egg Beaters	0
1 toasted whole-wheat English muffin	30
1 tsp. margarine	0
2 tsp. sugar-free jelly	0
1 c. pineapple cubes (in own juice)	20
coffee/tea with artificial sweetener	0
1 c. skim milk	12
TOTAL	**62**

Lunch

	Total Carbohydrate (g)
2 slices seven-grain bread	30
1/2 c. tuna fish (canned in water)	0
1 tbsp. reduced-fat mayonnaise	0
2 lettuce leaves	0
2 slices onion	0
2 1/2 c. watermelon	30
calorie-free beverage	0
TOTAL	**60**

Dinner

	Total Carbohydrate (g)
smothered pork chop	
4 oz. broiled pork chop (trim off fat)	0
1/4 c. defatted gravy	7
Hoppin' John	
1/2 c. cooked black-eyed peas	15
1/2 c. steamed white rice	20
1 1/2 c. cooked collard greens (no fat)	15
1 tsp. margarine	0
baked apple	
1 small baked apple (4 oz)	15
1 tsp. ground cinnamon	0
artificial sweetener	0
calorie-free beverage	0
TOTAL	**72**

Snack

	Total Carbohydrate (g)
finger sandwiches	
6 Triscuit® crackers	15
1 oz. cooked turkey (white meat)	0
calorie-free beverage	0
TOTAL	**15**

Day 4

Breakfast	Total Carbohydrate (g)
1 c. grits	30
3 oz. turkey sausage patty	0
1/2 oz. low-fat cheddar cheese	0
1 small Lender's® bagel (2 oz)	30
1 small orange (6 1/2 oz)	15
coffee/tea with artificial sweetener	0
2 tbsp. skim milk in coffee/tea	0
TOTAL	**75**

Lunch

	Total Carbohydrate (g)
1 c. chicken gumbo soup	
1 c. chicken broth	0
2 oz. broiled skinless chicken	0
1 c. cooked corn, onion, and okra	30
1 whole-wheat deli roll (1 oz)	15
tossed salad	
1 c. romaine and iceberg lettuce mix	5
1/4 c. chopped tomato	0
1/2 c. low-fat croutons	7
1 tbsp. French dressing	0
1 medium peach (6 oz)	15
calorie-free beverage	0
TOTAL	**72**

Dinner

	Total Carbohydrate (g)
4 oz. roasted turkey (white meat, without skin)	0
3/4 c. mashed potatoes	22
1/4 c. milk in mashed potatoes	3
1 1/2 c. cooked green beans	15
1 tsp. Margarine	0
1/2 cup cranberries	15
1/2 c. cornbread dressing	15
calorie-free beverage	0
TOTAL	**70**

Snack

	Total Carbohydrate (g)
trail mix	
3/4 oz. pretzels	15
10 peanuts	0
calorie-free beverage	0
TOTAL	**15**

Day 5

Breakfast	Total Carbohydrate (g)
1 medium corn muffin (2 oz.)	30
1 tsp. margarine	0
1/2 c. low-fat cottage cheese	3
1/2 c. canned peaches (in own juice)	15
coffee/tea with artificial sweetener	0
1 c. skim milk	12
TOTAL	**60**

Lunch

	Total Carbohydrate (g)
3 oz. grilled turkey burger	0
1 oz. low-fat cheddar cheese	0
1 whole-wheat bun (2 oz.)	30
1 cup cole slaw (prepared with low-fat mayo)	5
1 medium pear (4 oz.)	30
1/2 c. skim milk	6
TOTAL	**71**

Dinner

	Total Carbohydrate (g)
chicken and dumplings	
4 oz baked chicken (remove all skin)	0
2 dumplings (2"x 2" each)	30
1/4 c. defatted gravy	7
1/2 c. cooked carrots	5
1 tsp. margarine	0
1 c. sugar-free frozen yogurt	30
calorie-free beverage	0
TOTAL	**72**

Snack

	Total Carbohydrate (g)
3 graham crackers (2 1/2" square)	15
1/2 c. skim milk	6
calorie-free beverage	0
TOTAL	**21**

Day 6

Breakfast	Total Carbohydrate (g)
western omelet	
3 scrambled egg whites	0
1/2 c. cooked green peppers and onions	5
1 c. cooked grits	30
1 small biscuit (2 1/2" across)	15
1 tsp. margarine	0
17 small grapes (3 oz)	15
coffee/tea with artificial sweetener	0
2 tbsp. skim milk in coffee/tea	0
TOTAL	**65**

Lunch

	Total Carbohydrate (g)
2 slices rye bread	30
3 oz. sliced cooked roast beef	0
1 tsp. mayonnaise	0
1/2 cup potato salad (made with low-fat mayo)	15
1/2 c. fruit cocktail (in own juice)	15
1 c. skim milk	12
TOTAL	**72**

Dinner

	Total Carbohydrate (g)
4 oz. baked fresh lean ham	0
1 medium baked sweet potato (6 oz)	30
1 1/2 c. cooked turnip greens	15
1 small biscuit (2 1/2" across)	15
1 tsp. margarine	0
1/2 c. unsweetened applesauce	15
calorie-free beverage	0
TOTAL	**75**

Snack

	Total Carbohydrate (g)
nachos	
9 baked tortilla chips (1 oz)	15
1 oz. low-fat cheddar cheese	0
1/4 c. salsa	0
calorie-free beverage	0
TOTAL	**15**

Day 7

Breakfast	Total Carbohydrate (g)
4 pancakes (4" across)	30
2 tbsp. sugar-free maple syrup	0
3/4 c. vanilla low-fat yogurt	12
1 1/4 c. whole strawberries	15
coffee/tea with artificial sweetener	0
2 tbsp. skim milk in coffee/tea	0
TOTAL	**72**

Lunch

1 c. chili	
3 oz lean pan-broiled ground beef	0
1/2 c. tomato sauce	5
1/4 c. cooked green peppers	2
1/4 c. cooked onions	2
1/2 c. cooked kidney beans	15
2/3 c. steamed white rice	30
1/2 c. sugar-free vanilla ice cream	15
calorie-free beverage	0
TOTAL	**69**

Dinner

4 oz. blackened catfish	0
stewed tomatoes and okra	
1/2 c. cooked okra	5
1/4 c. stewed tomatoes	3
3/4 c. steamed brown rice	30
1 small biscuit (2 1/2" across)	15
1 tsp. margarine	0
1 c. cantaloupe melon cubes	15
calorie-free beverage	0
TOTAL	**68**

Snack

1 c. sugar-free pudding (made with skim milk)	12
calorie-free beverage	0
TOTAL	**12**

Appendix B
Food Diary

Sample Daily Food Diary

MEAL	FOOD CHOICE	SERVING SIZE	FOOD GROUP	CARB CHOICE	SMBG / COMMENTS	
					TIME	BG
BREAKFAST						
SNACK						
LUNCH						
SNACK						
DINNER						
SNACK						

Appendix C

Dictionary of Soul Food Terms

Ackee or **akee:** Introduced to Jamaica from Africa, ackee is a bright red fruit that is poisonous if eaten before fully mature. For this reason, ackee should never be forced open. When ripe, it will burst open to reveal three large black seeds and bright yellow flesh. Ackee and **salt fish** is the preferred breakfast of Jamaicans. Canned ackee can be found in West Indian markets.

Allspice: Called pimento in Jamaica, this berry the size of a large peppercorn has the taste of nutmeg, cinnamon, black pepper, and cloves.

Andouille: A Cajun sausage, lean and spicy, made of smoked pork. Used in **gumbos** and **jambalaya** dishes, it is also served grilled with red beans and rice.

Arrowroot: A neutral-tasting, easily digestible starch extracted from the root of tropical tubers. Arrowroot can be used instead of cornstarch as a glaze and to thicken sauces, puddings, and other foods.

Bammy: Jamaican **cassava** flatbread descended from the bread eaten by Jamaica's original inhabitants, the Arawak Indians.

Beans or **peas:** Interchangeable terms for red kidney beans (most popular), black beans, black-eyed peas, butter beans, lima and broad beans, pigeon peas, and yellow and green lentils. Beans are the West Indian Island's primary source of protein. Smaller peas are used for "rice and peas," and larger peas are used for stews and side dishes.

Beignet: Square French doughnut, deep-fried and dusted with powdered sugar.

Boudin or **black pudding:** A form of sausage, usually served fried, that may include pig's blood, thyme, and Scotch bonnet peppers. Boudin is frequently served with **souse**, a pork dish that can include any part of the pig. Authentic Cajun boudin is made with rice and spices.

Breadfruit: Related to the jackfruit, this is a large green fruit, usually about 10 inches in diameter, with a pebbly green skin and potato-like flesh. Breadfruit is picked and eaten before it ripens and is typically served like squash—baked, grilled, fried, boiled, or roasted after being stuffed with meat. It can also be thinly sliced and fried as chips.

Calabaza: A large yellow-skinned, pumpkin-like squash, also known as West Indian pumpkin. Used in island stews and vegetable dishes. Hubbard and butternut squash are similar in flavor and make the best substitutes.

Cajun cuisine: A French-southern style of cooking developed by French settlers in Louisiana, based on the use of rendered pork fat as cooking oil. Cajun cooking traditionally involved one large pot that served many.

Callaloo: A bitter-tasting, heart-shaped leaf of the taro plant, typically cooked like spinach and served with okra, onions, peppers, pork or ham, and shellfish. Like other greens, callaloo can be found both fresh and canned in West Indian markets.

Callaloo soup: A classic Caribbean soup made with **callaloo** leaves, fresh coconut milk, okra, yam, and sweet green peppers.

Carambola: Called star fruit or star apple, this oval, ribbed, orange-yellow fruit has a slightly sweet, acidic taste. When sliced in cross sections, it is star-shaped. Carambola can be used in desserts, as a garnish, in fruit salads, jellies, and preserves, or cooked with seafood.

Carossol: see **soursop.**

Cassava: A large, starchy tuber, also known as manioc or yucca. Sweet varieties are boiled and eaten as a vegetable. Bitter varieties contain a poison when raw and are used to make cassava bread (**bammy**), starch, and tapioca.

Chayote: Also known as christophine, cho-cho, and mirliton. A small vegetable in the squash family, shaped like a spiny, ridged pear with green to white skin and light green flesh. Chayote has a crisp, light taste, similar to a cucumber. It is used primarily as a side dish and can be eaten raw, stir-fried, steamed, or baked.

Chitterlings: More frequently called "chitlins," these are the small intestines of a pig. Chitlins can be purchased in most African American neighborhoods. They are usually cooked in a vinegared stock, after which they may be battered and fried.

Cho-cho: see **chayote.**

Christophine: see **chayote.**

Clabber: A thick, white liquid, not separated into curds and whey, that forms at the bottom when milk is allowed to stand. It is sour and similar to yogurt but different in flavor and texture. Traditionally in the South, clabber was used to make biscuits or sweetened with sugar and used as a beverage.

Coco: see **dasheen.**

Conch: A large spiral-shelled mollusk with edible and somewhat tough flesh. Before conch can be used in any recipe, it must be thoroughly beaten to tenderize it. Conch can be used in chowders, marinated for salads, or fried into spicy conch fritters.

Coo-coo or **cou-cou:** The Caribbean equivalent of polenta or grits. Once based on **cassava** or manioc meal, it is now made almost exclusively with cornmeal. Coo-coo can be baked, fried, or rolled into little balls and poached in soups or stews.

Crackling bread: A southern specialty of corn bread with **cracklings** mixed into the batter before baking. Also called "cracklin bread."

Cracklings: Also called "cracklins," these are crunchy pieces of pork or poultry fat after it has been rendered, or the crisp brown skin of fried or roasted pork. Cracklins are usually eaten as a snack.

Crawdads: see **crawfish.**

Crawfish: A freshwater crustacean, also known as crawdads or mudbugs, resembling a lobster without claws. Crawfish is served in various Louisiana dishes, such as **gumbo** and **étouffée**.

Creole Cuisine: Refers to the cooking of the French-speaking West Indies, Louisiana, and the Gulf States. This cooking style, which depends on butter as a basic fat, is a melding of ingredients and cooking methods from France, Spain, Africa, the Caribbean, and America.

Dandelion greens: The leaves of dandelions, these greens grow wild but are often grown in a hothouse for culinary use. Dandelion greens can be added to a pot of mixed greens or **gumbo**, tossed in a salad, or even made into wine.

Dasheen: Also known as coco, taro and tannia, dasheen is a starchy tuber with brown skin and bland-flavored, white flesh. It is usually served boiled or cut up and used as a thickener in hearty soups. Potatoes can be used as a substitute for dasheen in recipes.

Dirty rice: A Cajun-Creole dish, in which cooked long-grain rice is darkened with sautéed ground beef and pork, chicken livers, onions, celery, green peppers, parsley, and garlic.

Dhal: Hindi name for legumes, in the Caribbean it refers only to split peas or lentils.

Dressing: In Louisiana, dressing is synonymous with stuffing for poultry, fish, or meat.

It can be cooked separately or in the food into which it is stuffed. Dressing is usually well seasoned and based on corn bread, bread crumbs, or cubes of bread, although rice, potatoes, and other foods are also used.

Étouffée: Literally means "smothered." This Cajun stew is traditionally made with **crawfish** or shrimp, vegetables and a dark roux, cooked on low heat in a tightly closed pot with little or no liquid. Étouffée is usually served over rice.

Fatback: The clear fat from the back of a loin of pork. It may or may not be salt-cured. Fatback is used in many southern recipes. When it is rendered, fatback is called lard, and it is traditionally used as fat for frying chicken or fish.

Filé: A condiment of powdered, dried leaves of the sassafras tree, used to thicken and flavor **gumbo**.

Flor de Jamaica: A deep red flower that is dried and steeped in water to make a bright red drink with a slightly tart taste. Also known as sorrel or hibiscus, it is also used in jams and sauces. It is available dried and fresh during the Christmas season.

Gospel bird: Chicken was called "Gospel bird" because it was the traditional Sunday dinner. Although served at other meals, it is still referred to as "Gospel bird."

Guava or **guayaba:** A pear or plum-shaped fruit with pale yellow skin when ripe and white to pink flesh with many small, hard seeds. Guava has a strawberry-like taste and is used green or ripe in punches, syrups, jams, chutneys, and ice creams.

Gumbo: A Cajun-Creole soup or stew containing a variety of game, poultry, seafood, and vegetables, with okra or **filé** used for flavoring and thickening.

Head cheese: Not a cheese at all, but a jellied meat loaf made with pieces of meat from the head of a pig or a calf, onion, herbs, and seasonings. A gelatinous broth forms from the boiling, which is pickled. Head cheese is thinly sliced and usually served at room temperature. Also called "hog's head cheese," it is available in butchers' shops in African American neighborhoods.

Hibiscus: see **flor de Jamaica.**

Hoecake: see **johnnycake.**

Hog Maws: These are the stomach of the hog. A traditional southern dish, hog maws are often prepared with chitlins (**chitterlings**).

Hog's head cheese: see **head cheese.**

Hoppin' John: Said to have originated with African slaves on southern plantations, hoppin' John is a dish of black-eyed peas cooked with salt pork and seasonings and served with cooked rice. Tradition says that if hoppin' John is eaten on New Year's Day, it will bring good luck.

Igname: Similar in size and color to the potato but nuttier in flavor, this tuber should not be confused with the southern sweet yam or sweet potato. Caribbean yams are served boiled, mashed, baked, or as an ingredient of soups and stews.

Jambalaya: A highly spiced Cajun-Creole rice dish that may include ham, pork, sausage, shrimp, crawfish, beans, and other vegetables.

Johnnycake: Also called hoecake, and thought to be the precursor of the pancake, the johnnycake dates back to the early 1700s. It's a flat griddlecake made of cornmeal, salt, and either boiling water or cold milk. There is a Caribbean version made with flour. Today's johnnycakes often have eggs, oil or melted butter, and leavening (such as baking powder) added. Some versions are baked in the oven, more like traditional corn bread.

Malanga: Also called yautia, this tuber with white to pink flesh is a relative of **dasheen** or taro and is prevalent throughout the Caribbean. It is a natural thickener, used to thicken soups, stew, and bean dishes.

Manioc: see **cassava.**

Mamey apple: A large tropical fruit that yields edible, tangerine-colored pulp. With a flavor similar to a peach, mamey is often used to make jam.

Mirliton: see **chayote.**

Mudbugs: see **crawfish.**

Otaheite apple: The pear-shaped Otaheite apple, also known as a pomerac, ranges from pink to ruby red in color. Usually eaten fresh, it can also be packed in red wine or made into a cold drink.

Papaya: This fruit, native to South America, is still called a pawpaw by some Jamaicans. The papaya has an elongated, melon-like shape and is orange colored when ripe. Its bland flavor resembles that of a summer squash. Green papaya is used for chutneys or relishes and as a main dish when stuffed. When ripe, papaya is eaten like a melon or served in fruit salad. Papaya is also used as the basis for many commercial, natural meat tenderizers.

Passion fruit: An oval fruit with a tough shell whose color ranges from yellow to purple to deep chocolate. The golden yellow pulp is sweet, with a flavor like that of a peach. Passion fruit is used in juices, desserts, drinks, and sauces.

Pawpaw: see **papaya.**

Peas: see **beans.**

Pig's feet: Also known as trotters, these are the feet and ankles of a pig. Because they are bony and sinewy, pig's feet require long, slow cooking. Pig's feet are available pickled, fresh, and smoked. Southerners eat pig's feet with vinegar or hot sauce.

Pimento: see **allspice.**

Plantain: A green, fleshy fruit resembling the banana. Inedible raw, cooked plantains are served as appetizers or starchy side dishes in Caribbean cooking. Unripe plantains are green, ripe are yellow, and very ripe are dark. The ripeness determines how the plantain will be used. Green plantains are used for chips and stews, yellow plantains are used for mofongo (a Puerto Rican dish of mashed plantains, fried **pork rinds**, and garlic), and dark plantains are used for desserts.

Pomerac: see **Otaheite apple.**

Pork rinds: The crispy fried rinds of **fatback** that has been rendered into lard. They are available packaged in the South and in African American neighborhoods.

Pot likker (liquor): The vitamin-rich liquid left after cooking greens, vegetables, meat, etc. This broth is particularly popular in the southern United States and is traditionally served with corn bread or corn pone.

Praline: A confection of almonds or pecans boiled in a sugar mixture that hardens when cooled. Eighteenth-century Louisiana colonists changed the original recipe to utilize native pecans and brown sugar.

Roti: An Indian crêpe-like bread filled with curried meat, fish, chicken, or vegetables.

Roux: A slow-cooked, blended mixture of flour and melted fat or butter, used to add flavor and body to **gumbo** and other Cajun dishes.

Rutabaga: A turnip-like root vegetable with a strong taste, also called Swede turnips. It is usually yellow or orange in color.

Salt fish: Any fried, salted fish, but in the Caribbean, salt fish is most often cod.

Salt pork: A salt-cured belly cut of the hog with fat and streaks of lean, used primarily for flavoring and shortening. Also called "a streak a lean, streak a fat" salt pork is often confused with **fatback**.

Sorrel: see **flor de Jamaica.**

Soul food: Traditional African American food popular in the South. The term "soul food" is relatively new (circa 1960) and is thought to have derived from the cultural spirit and soul-satisfying flavors of black American food. Some of the dishes commonly thought of as soul food include ham hocks, grits, **chitterlings**, black-eyed peas, and collard greens.

Soursop: Also called carossol, the soursop is an elongated, spike-covered fruit with a white, creamy, lightly granular pulp. Soursop is usually eaten raw but is also used in drinks, punches, sherbets, and ice cream.

Souse meat: A jellied loaf or sausage made from pickled pig meat, it is the American variation on the souses of the Caribbean. Souse is frequently confused with **head cheese.** They are similar in ingredients and in taste.

Stamp and go: Spicy hot fritters made with salted codfish, popular throughout the Caribbean.

Star apple: see **carambola.**

Star fruit: see **carambola.**

Stuffing: see **dressing.**

Swede turnip: see **rutabaga.**

Tangelo: see **ugli.**

Tannia: see **dasheen.**

Taro: see **dasheen.**

Tasso: Thin-cut, lean strips of highly seasoned, marinated pork, which is heavily smoked. Used for seasoning in beans, **gumbos,** vegetables and many other Cajun dishes.

Trotters: see **pig's feet.**

Ugli: This hybrid citrus fruit created from grapefruit, orange, and tangerine, is often called tangelo. The ugli is lumpy, with a yellow skin usually served as juice or marmalade. It can also be glazed and dipped in chocolate.

West Indian pumpkin: see **calabaza.**

Yam: see **igname.**

Yautia: see **malanga.**

Yucca: see **cassava.**

About the Author

Constance Brown-Riggs is a nationally recognized nutritionist, registered dietitian, and certified diabetes educator with more than twenty-five years of experience in nutrition and dietetics. She is principal of CBR Nutrition Enterprises, located in Massapequa, New York.

Constance's work with *ESSENCE Magazine* as a nutrition consultant has given her a forum in which her views on nutrition, weight management, and healthy lifestyle can be read across the nation. She is frequently interviewed by *ESSENCE Magazine* for health-related stories, and she designed the personalized weight-loss meal plans for the health and fitness makeover participants in the *ESSENCE Total Makeover Book*, published January 2001. The participants' before-and-after pictures are proof of her belief that good nutrition is truly the best medicine. She was also the nutrition expert for *Lighten Up: The HealthQuest 30-day Weight-Loss Program*, published October 2001.

Constance is keenly aware of the need for culturally relevant educational tools and messages. She created the Diabetes Soul Food Pyramid with the goal of shortening the cultural distance between people with diabetes and their health-care providers. She is a past media spokesperson for the National Dairy Council's 20-City Minority Health Tour. When not conducting media interviews and consultations, Constance can be found in her office, providing individual consultation services for health maintenance and disease prevention and treatment, or marketing her Diabetes Soul Food Pyramid.

As a leader in her field, Constance has developed workshops and lectured on diabetes and other nutrition-related topics to organizations such as the American Dietetic Association, the New York State Dietetic Association, the American Academy of Physical Therapy and the University of South Carolina. She has also served as president of the New York State Dietetic Association, a 5,000-member organization.

Constance attended Queens College, Flushing, New York, completing her undergraduate and graduate studies, ultimately receiving a master's degree in nutrition education with honors for excellence in nutrition research.

Index

978-0-595-38051-0
0-595-38051-4

Breinigsville, PA USA
05 October 2009

225290BV00001B/11/A